Awaken Through Birth

From Fear to Power Through Evidence and Intuition

By Lauri Torgerson-White

www.awakenthrubirth.com

Copyright © 2023 Lauri Torgerson-White

All Rights Reserved.

Disclaimer: The advice in this book is not medical advice and may not be suitable for every birthing person or situation. This book does not serve as a substitute for the advice given by a medical professional and as such, any advice taken from this book should be discussed with your medical provider before implementation. This book is sold with the understanding that the author is not responsible for the individual birth experience after reading this book. While the author has used her best efforts in preparing this book, she makes no representations or warranties with respect to the accuracy or completeness of the contents of this book and specifically disclaims any implied warranties of merchantability or fitness for a particular purpose.

No part of this publication may be reproduced, distributed, or transmitted in any form or by any means, including photocopying, recording, or other electronic or mechanical methods, without the prior written permission of the author, except as permitted by U.S. copyright law.

ISBN 979-8-218-24318-0

Table of Contents

Gratitude	5
Preface	8
Part I	
Conversation 1: Through birth, you can unearth your power	15
Conversation 2: Why should you care?	20
Conversation 3: There is so much to learn about birth—but it's also so simple	24
Part II	
Conversation 4: What is unmedicated birth actually like?	37
Conversation 5: Two pink lines–now what?	47
Conversation 6: What are your greatest fears surrounding birth?	82
Part III	
Conversation 7: Tools of empowerment	103
Conversation 8: Envision your perfect birth experience	123
Part IV	
Conversation 9: My Birth Stories	138
Conversation 10: The power of presence postpartum	160
Recommended Resources to Learn More	167
References	169

To my beautiful children ~
Felix, Eliza, and Fletcher

Always remember that there are infinite possibilities in life, and you are capable of anything you truly desire.

I love you.

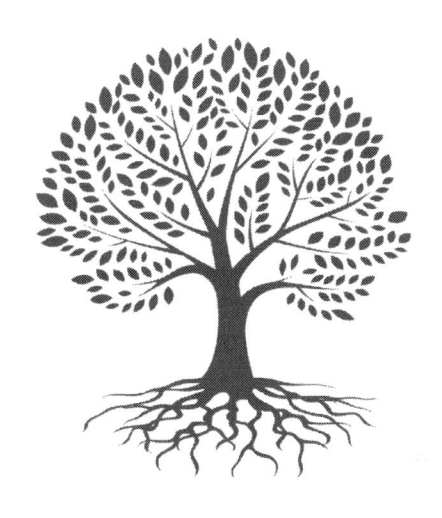

Gratitude

As with all things in life, beginning with gratitude feels the most generative to me. I would not exist and this book would not exist without so many others.

I have been passionate about birth from the moment I learned I was pregnant with my oldest child, Felix. That passion only grew as I went through my second pregnancy and birth with Eliza and my third pregnancy and birth with Fletcher. With that, I want to thank my three beautiful children, Felix, Eliza, and Fletcher for allowing me to be transformed as you each found solace and comfort in my womb and then took me through the adventures of birth. I want to thank you for making me a parent, for allowing me to make mistakes, and for inspiring me to awaken during birth and motherhood. This book would not exist without you. But more importantly, I would not be who I am today if I was not your mama. I love you all with everything that I am and ever will be.

It was during my third pregnancy that I decided to pursue birth work more seriously. I want to thank my midwife, Amy Lechtenberg, for allowing me to attend births with her and encouraging me in my journey. I have not yet figured out how to become a midwife while balancing work and motherhood, but it's still a dream of mine! The knowledge I gained working with you was essential to the writing of this book.

More recently, I was welcomed with open arms as a doula at Metro Detroit Doula Services. Thank you, Andrea Stainbrook and Amy Hammer, for letting me try to figure out how to work as a doula while also holding a full-time job! It was a rollercoaster of the very best kind, and the birth experience I gained undoubtedly influenced this book.

The stars aligned when I started working with Carmen Martinez Jover. You told me to write a book about birth and I did. Your confidence in this being my path gave me faith to pursue the unknown and for that I am forever grateful.

I want to thank Hillary Hendrickson. When you asked me to be your mentor during pregnancy, you helped me to trust that my knowledge is useful. I will forever cherish the conversations I had with you during your pregnancy (and what I think will be a lifelong friendship). Thank you so much for your thoughts on this book. Your edits definitely took it to the next level. I am so grateful for you.

I want to thank my mom, Cheryl Stephens, who birthed me and raised me. Through your own birth stories, you taught me that birth could be easy and fun. Through being you, you taught me that we should each be whoever we are (even if we like to veer off the beaten path!). Your love taught me to pursue whatever seemed interesting to me. Thank you. I love you.

I want to thank my dad, Tom Torgerson, for always believing in me as a writer. Your kind praise gave me the confidence I needed to start to write this book (even though you didn't know I was writing!). And during childhood, your love of fun taught me that life is an adventure. Thank you. I love you.

I want to thank my siblings (Shelley, Heidi, and Tommy Torgerson) who have been my lifelong, built-in friends and supports. I won the jackpot with my family. I don't know what I would do without you. I love you all so much.

Last, but certainly not least, I want to thank my best friend, never-ending supporter, and partner in the adventures of life—my husband, Ryan White. You have always believed in me even more than I believe in myself. I would not be the person I am today without what truly feels like unconditional love and unfaltering support. This book would not have happened without you. Our family would not be what it is without you. My gratitude for you overflows every day of our lives. I love you forever and ever.

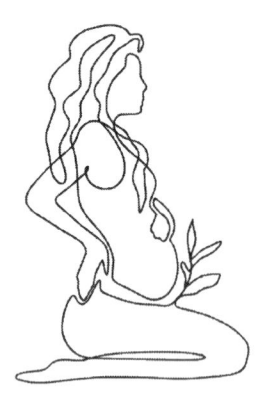

Preface

I am not your average birth expert. I am not a midwife or a doctor. While I have worked as a doula in the past, right now I work as a research biologist studying the inner lives of animals. But I have a secret that I can't hold in anymore. You may or may not think I have the credentials necessary to share it, but I must share it all the same. I know the potential birth can have in your life because I have gone through three births of my own, each resulting in a beautiful child and a transformation of my soul. With that, this book is not your average book about birth. I am not here to tell you what to do or how to birth. It would be presumptuous of me to do so. I don't know you and I don't know your circumstances. Instead, I will share knowledge, both from my own lived experience and from scientific research, that will empower you to decide for yourself how you want to birth.

Birth can transform you and be the dawn of a journey towards higher consciousness.

While this knowledge of potential transformation cannot be fully explained by science, the reality is that many of the tools that will lead you to this transformation are based in science. As a researcher, I am skilled at uncovering, understanding, and distilling this research in a way that will allow you to get closer to a transformation of your soul, if you so choose.

I'd love to do you the favor of summarizing all of the information I've gained in the years of being pregnant, having babies, being a mother, learning about birth on my journey to becoming a doula, and honestly, being a spiritual seeker. There is a reality out there where birth transforms and empowers you, and I'd like to take you straight there rather than letting you stop off at the exits where birth is dangerous and painful or, even worse, allowing you to experience birth as traumatic before getting to the empowering birth you so desire.

This book is constructed differently than most books. I want it to be a conversation between you and me. I want to use the power of storytelling to help you learn. There are times that I may gloss over some of the details of the actual physical mechanics of birth. With that, I start here by giving you some general information about how birth works. Throughout the book I'll talk about your cervix, dilation, and stages of labor. Here are some definitions to guide your learning.

The basics of birth

- Your uterus is the organ that houses your baby. The opening of your uterus, that connects to your vagina, is called the cervix.
- Within your uterus, your baby is attached via an umbilical cord to your placenta. The placenta is an organ that your body created to nourish your baby and attaches to the wall of your uterus.
- Contractions are the tightening of your uterine muscles. That tightening opens (dilates) your cervix and allows your baby to be born. Some people call contractions "waves," "surges," or "cramps."
- Dilation refers to the size of the opening of your cervix (the neck-like opening of your uterus). Your cervix will be open 10 cm when your baby emerges.
- Effacement refers to the thinning and shortening of your cervix. Your cervix will be 100% effaced when your baby is born.
- Early labor begins when your contractions begin and ends when your cervix is 6 cm dilated.
- Active labor begins when your cervix is 6 cm dilated and ends when your cervix is 10 cm dilated.
- The pushing phase (also known as the second stage of labor) begins when your cervix is 10 cm dilated and ends with a baby in your arms.
- The third stage of labor begins immediately after your baby is born and ends when you birth your beautiful, amazing placenta (that magical organ you created to nourish your baby).

List of Acronyms

- ACOG: The American College of Obstetricians and Gynecologists
- CNM: Certified Nurse Midwife
- CPM: Certified Professional Midwife
- DEM: Direct-Entry Midwife
- OB-GYN: Obstetrician/Gynecologist

Aiming for inclusivity

Throughout the book, I refer to birthing people as "women" in places where the research I cite is based on cisgender women or in places where I, as a cisgender woman myself, am referring to the experiences that I know other cisgender women have. In other places, I use more inclusive language. While I talk about the impact of the patriarchy on women specifically, I recognize that all minoritized groups have been impacted by the patriarchal nature of society. Transgender men and nonbinary people also give birth and I support all of you in finding your power through birth. Much of this book is based on research in "women," possibly because nonbinary and transgender were not options on the demographic forms filled out by study participants. Regardless of the research or society's view that birth is something experienced only by cisgender women, I genuinely hope birth can empower all of you, no matter what your gender identity.

This book is written from an American perspective, with many of the cited statistics coming from the United States. I describe the American maternal health care system and home birth in the United States because this is the system I know best. That said, there are many countries in the world that approach birth more holistically than happens in the United States. And there are others that don't. Regardless of where in the world you are, you deserve to be empowered by birth and I believe there are many tools in this book that can help you get there.

Additionally, there are times when I refer to a "partner." I don't want this to turn any single parents away. I am supportive of all types of families and recognize that single parenting is tough enough, without having to live in a society set up for dual-parent households. Finally, while I highly encourage you to hire a doula, I recognize that can be financially out of reach for some. I did not have a doula myself, so while doulas are so helpful, they aren't essential if you are willing to do the work to prepare. Please know that, even without a doula or a partner, you can find your power, and when you do, you'll truly be ready to change the world because you did it all on your own!

What to expect from this book

This book is structured in four parts, each of which contains what I like to think of as one or more Conversations between you and me. You can think of each Conversation as a chapter if you'd like, but when I was writing them, I felt like I was in conversation with you. In Part I, we'll explore why you should care about birth, explore how your mind creates your birth experience, and dive into the possibilities for empowerment that you may not know exist. In Part II, we will get into the nitty gritty of birth. In Conversation 4, through storytelling, we will learn what unmedicated birth can look like. Conversation 5 is designed to help you choose your birthing location and provider and does a deep dive into the questions you can ask your provider to be sure that they will be supportive of the birth you aim to create. Conversation 6 is extremely useful for those of you who are coming to birth with fears. I ask the questions that so many are afraid to explore, and through that, begin to dissolve your fears through education, which is the first step to having an awakened birth. Part III prepares you for birth by providing you with "tools of empowerment" and guiding you through a process to envision your ideal birth and create a birth plan. Finally, Part IV uses my own stories to help you see that birth and the early postpartum days can be a time of power, transformation, joy, and awakening.

  I recommend you keep a journal by your side while you are reading. Take note of what grabs your attention and what resonates with you. This will be helpful in digging deep into your fears and desires surrounding birth. When we get to Conversation 7, I'll suggest more journal prompts that will allow you to prepare for an awakened birth.

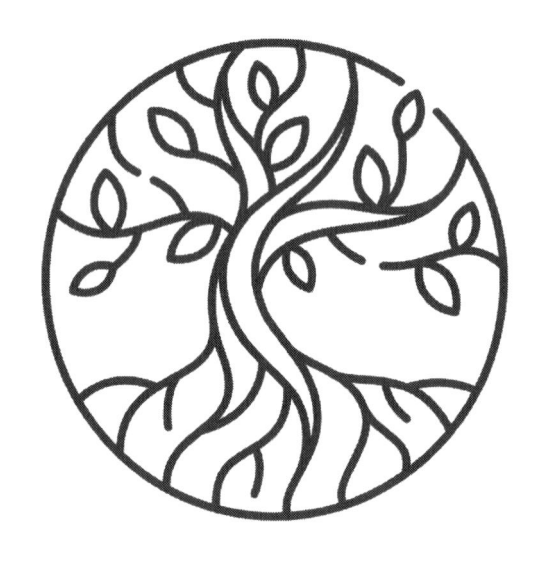

I

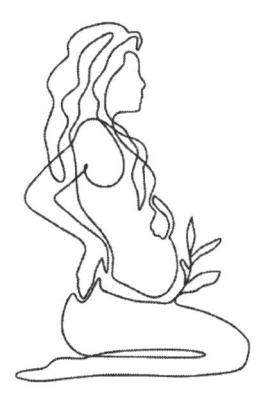

Conversation 1

Through birth, you can unearth your power

You are probably used to having your power taken from you, or dare I say, handing that power over to men, your parents, your boss, the government, or "name your favorite authority figure here." You have been taught not to trust your inner knowing. And so, you have silenced that inner voice over and over again—probably without even realizing it. Even though you work hard daily and put everything you have into whatever you're doing, you may have told yourself that you didn't deserve that promotion or raise or time for self-care, and so you didn't advocate for yourself. Or you've allowed others to treat you in ways that you knew were wrong, maybe taking credit for your ideas or accomplishments, but you made excuses because, doesn't every woman get treated in that way? We've all been victims in our lives, and for some the conditions make it especially hard to shift away from victimhood to power. But, birth is not the time to silence your inner knowing, to be a victim, and to give your power away. Birth is the time to go deep into your core, find your physical strength, and with that unearth the power that you hold but have kept buried.

It's ironic that the time when you're most vulnerable, when it's easiest to become a victim, is also the perfect time to take back our power. Once you become a parent, you will likely find yourself willing to do *anything* to create a world where your child can thrive. If you are having your babies biologically, I believe that begins the moment you decide to care for that being forming inside of you. Let's use that mama bear instinct to reclaim your power and transform.

This book will be a combination of evidence-based research on birth, (I am, after all, a scientist) with smatterings of my own intuitive knowing. Much of what happens during birth is beyond the scope of science, yet is no less based in reality. I urge you to read with an open mind, take what feels right to you, and leave the rest. There is no one right way to navigate birth. There is only the way that is right for you and your child, and my goal with this book is to help you find the path that empowers and transforms you.

Choosing our experience

The stories society tells us about birth are filled with lies. But because I believe in the good of humanity, I do not believe that they are purposeful lies. But, they are lies all the same. You've all seen it: the image of the beet-red woman, sweaty hair, feet in stirrups, screaming like someone is using a corkscrew to rip her baby out of her body. Unfortunately, this image becomes the reality for so many because the mind-body connection is strong. Science has not fully caught up with what many of us can vouch for, even if only anecdotally, but there IS emerging science in support of this assertion. Our mind creates our experience, and this is just as true while we are bringing new life into this world as it is when we allow ourselves to be upset by a traffic jam. We could just as easily take that time in the traffic jam to listen to our favorite music, to call a friend we haven't talked to in years, or to simply be in the beautiful sunshine. But many of us choose to emotionally suffer when our bodies are stuck in a traffic jam. Right? Think back to the last time you were stuck in traffic. Remember how your shoulders and jaw tensed up. You started tapping your fingers impatiently. You chose to suffer because society told you that life must happen in a hurry—and the traffic jam is slowing down that plan.

In the same way, when our bodies are bringing new life into this world, many of us experience suffering that has been conditioned into us by doctors, that friend with the horrifying birth story, movies and TV shows, and the media. But, listen to this: Neither suffering in a traffic jam nor while our babies enter the world is the only path we can take. We don't have to suffer! But suffering is the path we've learned and I want to disrupt that for you.

Now, I recognize that I'm comparing sitting in a car to having another human emerge from your vagina, which seems silly, but if our minds can create suffering for no good reason while we sit in a car, could our minds also create joy and empowerment when we bring new life into the world? I think so.

My birth experiences were intense. During birth, I am viscerally in my body, while also experiencing something out of body. While I vacillate between calm focus and feeling completely out of control during my births, I am continuously in awe of the unbridled strength of my uterine muscles. And for me, awe is the connection to the divine, to Mother Earth, to God, to the Universe, to nature, or to "whatever you choose to call that something bigger than ourselves," and hence, to my power. If it is hard for you to believe in something bigger than yourself, that's okay—feel free to ignore those references throughout the book. Everything I'm saying applies to YOU and YOUR BABY no matter what your spiritual beliefs are.

When my mind wanders back to the birth of my children, my memories of birth are devoid of suffering. I remember birth as transformative. I remember birth as the moment in my life when I was most IN MY POWER, to my very core, quite literally. I remember birth with joy and love and longing and sometimes tears shed at the idea of never experiencing that high again, but also deep gratitude that the stars aligned for me in a way that allowed birth to transform me. While we've been told that we forget the pain of birth so that we can do it again, for me, this rosy view of birth arose immediately after my babies each joined us earthside. (Ask my husband if you don't believe me!) Just as my children came through birth to enter a new realm on earth, I emerged through birth *with* my children to enter a new reality for me, a reality where I stand more fully in my power. And I now have that power forever. I am always able to look back on my birth experiences and know that, if I could do that with such power and strength, I can do absolutely anything.

Birth (as well as parenting—we'll go there later) has the power to destroy or to empower and transform. For you and for your child, I want to help you find the pathway that leads to power and transformation. That is why I am writing this book.

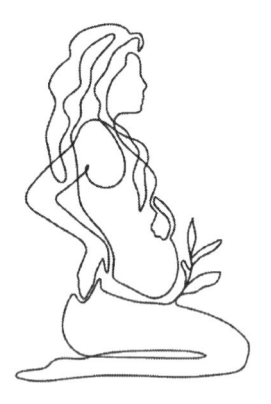

Conversation 2

Why should you care?

You might be wondering why you should care. Perhaps your plan is to get an elective cesarean section or to schedule an induction with an epidural and watch reality TV as your contractions pass through, unnoticed except for what you see on the bedside monitor. While I firmly believe that each person should make their own choices regarding birth, and both an epidural and an elective cesarean can be the right choice, I also know that surprises are a part of birth, and I don't want you to be surprised and unable to cope (let alone thrive) if your plans are disrupted by complications that could be traumatic. Perhaps you think you are already prepared. After all, you are a human hoping to have a baby, and haven't billions of others come before you? As we talked about in Conversation 1, the reality is that society has prepared you to have a highly medicalized birth that may leave you feeling somewhat underwhelmed at best, traumatized at worst. This book is here to help you undo the conditioning that society has instilled in you so that you can get back to nature and birth your baby as the empowered goddess we all know you are.

Birth sticks with you, so let's make it good!

Just as empowerment through birth is real, so too is birth trauma.[1] For mothers who have gone through it, it can evoke intense suffering long after their babies leave their diapers behind. It can leave us feeling taken advantage of and powerless. Indeed, about a third of women experience traumatic births[2] and up to 6% of women develop post-traumatic stress disorder (PTSD) as a result of going through childbirth.[3-6] Yes, that's the same psychological disorder that commonly develops among soldiers, breast cancer survivors, and refugees.[7-9] So even if you aren't interested in becoming empowered by birth (or you think I'm completely ridiculous in suggesting that as a possibility), keep reading, because I'd like at the very least to stop you from being hurt by birth trauma.

What about your baby? Most of us believe that, because we don't remember our own births, there's no way that babies could be impacted by a traumatic entry into this world. Well, first off, if you're planning on breastfeeding, you should know that birth trauma can impact the breastfeeding relationship.[2] Research has demonstrated that longer and more difficult labors, vacuum extraction of baby, and unexpected cesarean all resulted in a more difficult breastfeeding journey.[10–13] Women who had traumatic births have reported suffering uncontrollable flashbacks and low milk supplies that negatively impacted their breastfeeding relationship.[2] Beyond breastfeeding, birth trauma can impact your confidence in your ability to parent and can make it harder to develop a secure attachment to your baby.[14] We know that mothers remember and are impacted by birth trauma and through those memories, babies are too. But can the traumatic experience of birth impact the baby directly?

Recent research suggests that the trauma from our own births can impact the way we cope in the world. Indeed, complications during birth have been associated with increased rates of depression and anxiety during childhood.[15,16] In seven-year old children who were born early, those who had experienced more neonatal complications perceived pain from a blood draw to be more severe than those who had fewer.[17] There are recorded accounts of very young children who have never been told about their own births, but who recount details that they could not have known except through memory. There are even accounts of adults who are taken back to birth memories via hypnosis.[18] While I can't offer hard and fast evidence that conscious birth memories can impact our children, I also can't prove that those memories aren't hidden somewhere deep in our childrens' subconscious brains. I'd prefer to help you play it safe by working to ensure the calmest entry for your child into this world.

Our children need the best start they can get

I believe we are at a tipping point in human consciousness. Whether you believe this or not is irrelevant. All around us, we see suffering in the form of natural disasters, war, intolerance, racism, sexism, bullying, and gun violence. Yet, I also see a growing trend in spiritual seeking, in attempting to connect to something bigger than ourselves. My hope is that this next generation, OUR children, can change the course of humanity. They are our hope. They can take the love that I know permeates through all beings on earth and amplify that love. But to do that, they need access to that love, and I believe that coming into the earth in a gentle, loving way will give them the head start they need. It isn't the only pathway, but it's a powerful one! As our children literally squeeze through our bodies to become change agents in the world, we can empower them by empowering ourselves. That is what birth can do.

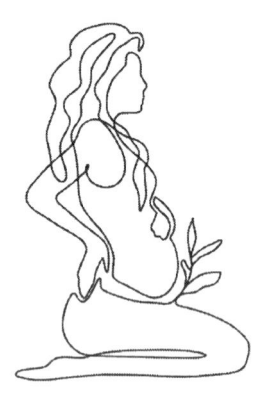

Conversation 3

There is so much to learn about birth—but it's also so simple

Let me take you back to 2011, to the moment I learned I was pregnant with my oldest. My husband, Ryan, and I were staying in a motel with our dog, Izze, while visiting a friend from graduate school. My period was a few days late, and we were planning on enjoying a few alcoholic beverages, so I decided to take a pregnancy test, just in case. We'd been married for about three weeks and I thought that the chances of a positive test were almost nil, but wanted to be careful. I sat in the Howard Johnson bathroom peeing on a stick while Ryan waited anxiously with our dog just outside the door. Just as the second pink line showed up and I started to yell to Ryan, "I'M PREGNANT!", our dog began to poop on the floor. Cue scene to Ryan frantically carrying our five pound pom-chi out of the room with poop hanging from her butt while I ran after him waving the positive test in the air.

Once we recovered from shock (and cleaned up the poop), we immediately went to the store where I purchased a jar of prenatal vitamins, a candy bar, and the book, *What to Expect When You're Expecting*. Like most, I had a million questions about the new life growing in my body, and I immediately started looking for answers. I'll never forget laying in bed that night eating my candy bar, eyes wide open in disbelief as I sought answers to my questions. I then spent the next eight months (and two subsequent pregnancies plus a journey to becoming a birth doula) taking in every snippet of information I could about birth. While much of what I took in was evidence-based, much was also driven by the fear that plagues our culture in a society that has medicalized birth.

Stepping outside of the fear-based birth model

The horror stories we hear about hospital births seem to be running rampant through society right now. From unwanted cesareans to failed inductions to threats that your baby will die if you don't do what the doctor says, a culture of fear has been created around birth. And dare I say that culture is being perpetuated not only by the practices that have become commonplace during hospital births, but also by the natural birth crowd who is desperately trying to save women from what they perceive as horrific hospital births. As with most things in 21st century America, birth is often

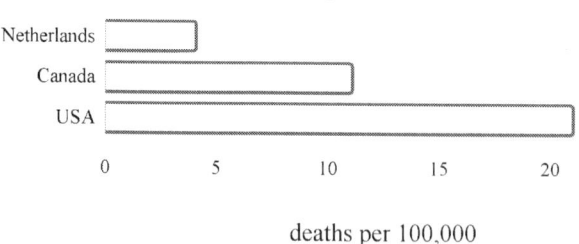

Figure 1: Maternal Mortality Rates

Country	deaths per 100,000
Netherlands	~4
Canada	~11
USA	~21

perceived in black and white, with advocates for each side (hospital birth vs. home birth) sometimes vilifying the other side. The reality has many shades of gray.

There are other places in the world where these two sides come together and work as a team,[19] and in those countries, maternal and neonatal health outcomes are significantly better. For example, while 21 out of 100,000 women die during childbirth in the United States, that number is only 11 out of 100,000 in Canada and 4 out of 100,000 in the Netherlands (which coincidentally also has the highest rate of home births–see figure 1).[20] When you consider the annual number of births in the United States, that means that hundreds of women are dying unnecessarily,[21] with a disproportionate number of those being women of color.[22] The Netherlands and Canada both have maternal health models where low-risk women can choose to have their babies at home and where midwives and physicians work together.[23] We need to merge the traditional midwifery model whereby birth is considered to be a natural physiological process with the Western medical model whereby surgeons are ready to step in if an emergency should arise.

While fear can result from the practices seen in hospitals, fear also runs deep in the medical professionals attending births in the medical establishment.[24] Fear has been woven into the system. Having been taught that birth is a medical condition, to mitigate the problems that can (but rarely do) arise during birth, their education has been focused largely on controlling the birthing process through Western medical ways. Interventions often lead to more interventions. First, an epidural is given to mitigate pain. Then, Pitocin might be added to speed birth along after the epidural slows things down. Finally, a cesarean section may be recommended if your baby's in distress from the Pitocin causing your uterus to contract unnaturally frequently and strongly.[25,26] Of course, it doesn't always play out this way, but the research suggests that each intervention heightens the risk of the next intervention. The doctors and nurses are trying to get your baby to you in the *best way they know how*. Let me repeat, they are doing the best they can with the information and training they have. These individuals are not to blame.

Instead, the system that raised and educated them is flawed. The American medical system is profit-driven and the risk of malpractice litigation is very real. Indeed, research suggests that both profits and fear of litigation impact cesarean rates.[27] Most American hospitals are private non-profit, but ironically these institutions generate massive profits, with the average CEO making upwards of $3.5 million per year and the top 82 hospitals making more than $200 billion in profits.[28,29] Because cesareans cost $12,000 more than vaginal birth,[30] you'd expect to see a correlation between hospital profits and the number of cesareans performed in a hospital and indeed, hospitals that make the most profit also perform the most cesareans.[31] Furthermore, the risk of malpractice lawsuits against physicians and hospitals creates fear that leads doctors (likely subconsciously) to recommend cesareans when they may not be medically necessary.[32] Of course, there are times when I thank the Universe for Western medicine, times when a cesarean is absolutely the only way to save a baby's or a parent's life. I am eternally grateful at those times. But at a time when the World Health Organization recommends a cesarean rate of no more than 15%,[33] it is essential that we look at the fear that is driving the 32% cesarean rate in the United States.

This is not the only way. Together, we can use knowledge to empower rather than to create fear. I want you to combine the information in this book with your inner knowing to manifest the sort of birth that rocks you to your very core in the best of ways.

Into a new (old!) birth paradigm

Pain doesn't always have to be pain; it can be immense strength

While I have dabbled in birth for over a decade as a mother, a doula, and through attending home births in an attempt at beginning a midwifery apprenticeship (which is still a goal that I haven't figured out how to achieve while also supporting my family financially), by day I'm a biologist, specifically, an animal behavior and welfare scientist. Given this background, I know that the ability to reproduce and pass on our genes is the very basis for natural selection and evolution. Scientists call it fitness; animals who have more healthy offspring have higher fitness, which means that their genes are more likely to be more prevalent in the next generation. Over many generations, species evolve. As a species that usually only has one baby at a time, it would not be adaptive for birth to be as painful as the movies make it seem because then WE'D NEVER DO IT AGAIN! We would not pass on our genes and eventually, we'd go extinct. Cue the doomsday soundtrack!

Birth is a natural physiological process and what we call labor pain is usually quite different from the pain associated with acute injury or illness. In layperson's terms, pushing a baby out of a birth canal that was meant to birth your baby is not the same as breaking a bone. What we call pain during childbirth is natural, purposeful, productive, and something you can prepare for.[34] What many people call "pain" can be reimagined as "power." You're a portal from whatever is on the other side–that seems pretty powerful to me!

The sensations associated with birth don't have to be painful. Repeat that out loud because you're probably thinking I've lost my mind. Birth does not have to be painful. Now yell it: "BIRTH DOES NOT HAVE TO BE PAINFUL!" Pain, like all sensations, is a construct of our minds,[35] and when we believe we are in pain, we will be in pain. Have you ever seen an animal give birth? When I was pregnant with my second child, in a (successful) attempt to dispel fear, I spent a lot of time watching videos of animals giving birth. And guess what? When a giraffe gives birth, she doesn't scream. Honestly, she doesn't even appear all that uncomfortable. No one is there to give her pain medications, because why would Mother Earth/God/the Universe (or evolution for those of you who are more science-minded) make birth a painful process?

Let's shift our thinking: instead of pain, think pressure. And when you feel intense pressure, think POWER.

The strength of your uterus is going to blow your mind!

Your uterine muscles are going to make you feel like the most amazing body builder. Have you ever seen those bodybuilding competitions where the men have insanely large muscles and are lifting giant barbells? Or maybe you've seen those log rolling competitions with the lumberjacks in flannel shirts? That's you, except for you're even more powerful because your uterine muscles are able to work involuntarily. Unlike the body builder, you don't need to use willpower to lift the barbell. Instead, your muscles know exactly how to contract to gently, but POWERFULLY, move your baby into your birth canal and into the world. You just get to ride the waves of your insanely powerful muscles.

The power of your uterine muscles is like nothing you have ever experienced. If you aren't prepared, it will take you by surprise and you may even mistake that power, and the downward pressure that results from those muscles pushing your baby out, as pain. I am not here to mislead you and tell you that birth is easy. There's a reason people call it labor. There were times in all three of my births that I wanted to give up. Despite my intention to birth my first child unmedicated, once those surges hit, I swore I would get a cesarean the second I arrived at the hospital. (But Felix was born vaginally after an intense 2-hour birth; I'll share my birth stories at the end of the book.) Birth is hard work! You should be training for it, just as you'd train for any physical event. I want you to learn how to harness the power of your mind to go inward during the birth process, marvel at the power of your body, and allow your baby to come earthside through a portal that is filled with calm-inducing hormones like oxytocin rather than fight-or-flight inducing hormones like epinephrine.

Our bodies are perfectly adapted to birth our babies

Your uterus has two sets of muscles that work together to birth your baby. The outer layer runs longitudinally while the inner layer is a series of circles that go around the uterus horizontally. The inner layer contracts during pregnancy to hug your baby and keep them safe inside of you. But during birth, that inner layer relaxes and the outer layer contracts and pulls open those inner muscles that have been holding your cervix closed, thus dilating your cervix and making room for baby to come through. When your baby and your body have decided that it is time for baby to come earthside, those amazing uterine muscles work together to squeeze your baby out through your vagina. They can even work together to bring your baby into the world if you're completely unaware. Doctors call this the "fetal ejection reflex." This sounds a bit like a baby cannon to me, but it's amazing all the same. There are reports of women in comas and even women without brain activity delivering their babies vaginally in this way.[36] Let that sit with you for a minute. If you allowed your body to take over and your conscious mind to take a backseat, your baby would come peacefully into the world. If that doesn't sound like the Universe working through us, like love permeating our bodies to bring our babies earthside, I don't know what does.

You control your mind—your mind doesn't control you

I'm closing my eyes right now. Well yes, not exactly now because I can't type with my eyes closed but…pausing and closing my eyes. I want you to close your eyes too for a moment and feel the tingling in your hands. I'll wait while you do that. Slowly count to ten while you notice that tingling.

Okay, are you back? Notice how when you focus on the feeling of your hands, the other sensations in your body seem less noticeable. Go ahead and try again. I'll wait. While your consciousness is directed at your hands, you aren't as focused on other sensations in your body. If there are other sensations, you can notice them without judging them as good or bad. I've tested this before when I've had a sore neck or back, and guess what? I'm able to more easily be with the sensation in my neck or back by focusing my attention elsewhere in my body. I can accept that sensation without judgment, which allows me to release any suffering attached to that sensation. You can do this with the physical sensations of birth. But what about emotions? Can this work to release fear? It can. I've tested this when I was overcome by the fear of public speaking. I once had to unexpectedly speak on a panel, with no time for preparation. After a lifetime of being terrified of public speaking, I sat on-stage in front of an auditorium full of people and focused my attention on the tingling sensation of my feet instead of the fear coursing through my veins. The result: I was told after the panel that I spoke like a "marketing genius."

Throughout your pregnancy, I'd like you to try this any time you feel physical or emotional discomfort, fear, or anxiety. This practice will prepare you to ride the waves that will bring your baby closer to you and eventually, into your arms. Notice how I call them "waves" instead of "contractions." That is because words have power. Remember that old saying "sticks and stones can break my bones but words can never hurt me"? I want you to erase that from your memory. Words can take your power away.

Words create reality

We will get into this a bit more later, but I want you to start to get comfortable with the idea that words create your reality. When you call a sensation "pain," it becomes pain. With practice, if you call a sensation "pressure," it becomes pressure and the fear that we associate with pain is released. It's that simple.

Evidence for the mind-body connection

A variety of psychological processes impact our perception of pain.[37] As I noted earlier, placing our attention away from pain can allow us to be less judgmental about that sensation.[38] Alternatively, focusing our attention on what we think is causing us pain and calling it pain can increase our pain perception. Our thinking surrounding pain impacts our perception. If we attend to the sensations of birth without judgment, we will experience them differently than if we judge them in the negative light of pain. If we believe birth is painful, it very likely will be. If we expect birth to be short and instead it is long, we will likely experience more pain as the hours pass. We catastrophize our pain by imagining how absolutely horrible it will be, and with that, we significantly worsen our pain experience.[39–42] Fear, anxiety, and distress increase pain while positive emotions can decrease pain.[43–46]

Science tells us that our mind impacts our pain experience.[37,47] In one study, participants held onto a very cold (freezer temperature) rod for a short amount of time and were asked to rate their pain.[48] The scientists varied the color of the rod (red versus blue) and whether the participant looked at or away from the rod. Even though the temperature of the rod and the amount of time that the rod was held did not vary, the experience of pain varied significantly across these experimental conditions. The red rod resulted in more intense and unpleasant pain than the blue rod, and the experience of pain became even more intense and unpleasant when the participant looked at instead of away from the rod. In another example, patients with fibromyalgia (a chronic pain disorder) who were poked experienced less pain when they were with their significant others than when they were alone.[49,50] This mind-body connection is particularly relevant during childbirth, a time when women who expect more pain also experience more pain.[51,52] Research demonstrates that women with severe fear of childbirth experience significantly higher levels of pain than those without fear, with the mother's mental health playing a role in that experience.[53]

Now that you understand the importance of untangling your fears in having an awakened birth, let's get started by first learning what your average, unmedicated birth might look like.

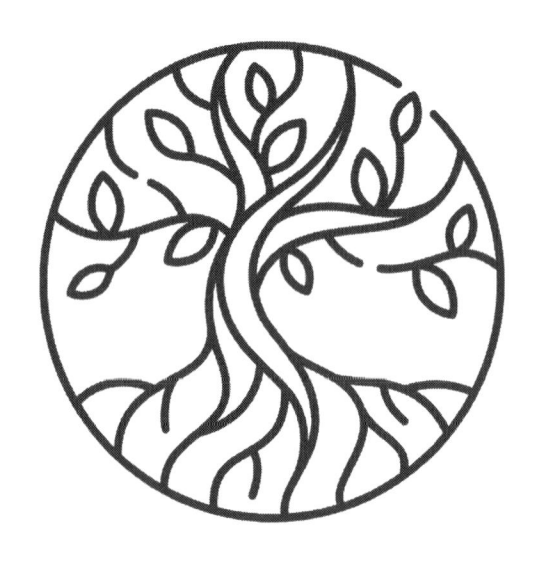

II

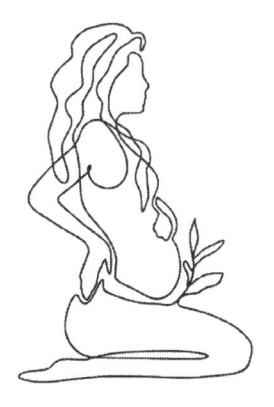

Conversation 4

What is unmedicated birth actually like?

Fear is incomplete knowledge. –Agatha Christie

Have you ever heard the saying, "knowledge is power"? Take that to heart, because only once you know better, can you do better. I have been curious from the time I was born. It's why I'm a scientist and why I'm a spiritual seeker and why I'm sort of obsessed with self-development, all because I'm learning more. But many of us are so afraid of birth that we choose not to learn and instead, to let someone else dictate what happens to us during pregnancy, birth, and beyond. It often feels easier to blindly trust our medical providers, especially because we are told that they know what is best. While their knowledge is extremely valuable when complications arise during birth, I firmly believe you should know what you're getting into. You likely wouldn't run a marathon without knowing how long the race is and preparing yourself for how you'll cope when you hit the wall. So why would you go into birth not knowing what it is like? Before we dive into common fears surrounding birth, I want to provide you with what I think is a digestible, bite-size amount of information that will prepare you for birth. What does unmedicated, physiological birth look like?

While you can read online, in a clinical way, about the stages of labor, I'd prefer to tell you about birth with a story. You are the main character. The following story will depict a home birth rather than a hospital. This is not to say that you must or even should have a home birth. Instead, I choose home here because an unmedicated, physiological birth is most likely to unfold as nature intended in a safe space where medical interventions are offered at an absolute minimum. You might feel safest in a hospital, and if that's the case, you should have your baby there. But for now, I'd like you to open your mind to all possibilities. You can narrow them as you read through this book. This is what an unmedicated, physiological birth often looks like:

Early labor

You went to bed early last night because your stomach feels like it just cannot get any bigger, and you know that you'll wake up a million times and have to hang onto the headboard to leverage your strength in a way that can allow you to change sides. You can't wait for a time when you can lay on your back again. (You've been laying on your side since the second trimester so as not to put pressure on the blood supply that goes to your baby.) When you wake up and look at the clock, it's 3:33 AM, and you feel a bit different from usual. A bit restless, even. But you still have three hours until your alarm, so you switch sides, close your eyes, and try to go back to sleep. As your mind races, thinking about all the things you still need to do before baby comes, you notice a crampy feeling in your lower abdomen. It feels just like period cramps, and you wonder if it's the extra hot sauce you put on everything lately causing your intestines to scream at you. You get out of bed and go to the bathroom and when you sit down, your lower abdomen feels crampy again. If you weren't almost 40 weeks pregnant, you'd swear that your period was going to start any minute with these cramps. And then it hits you, crap, you're almost 40 weeks pregnant and you feel crampy. Maybe this is labor? Given how mild the cramping is, you're unsure. So you go and get back in bed and try to go back to sleep.

As you lie there thinking about the things you'll do tomorrow after work: your grocery list, laundry, wash baby clothes…your mind also wanders to your very near future. You wonder what kind of parent you'll be and whether your partner will be a good parent. And then you feel crampy again. This time, you're more awake and more aware, and so you feel your belly and it's hardening, the same way it's been hardening on and off for a few weeks with Braxton Hicks contractions. But this time, it isn't only your belly hardening, but also your lower belly feeling slightly crampy. At this point, it's now 4:30 AM, which means you've had three crampy feelings in about an hour. Your doula has been telling you all along that you need to try to rest as much as possible when you're in early labor, and given this might be early labor, you put on a sleep story and close your eyes. Miraculously, you're able to drift off to sleep…

Your alarm jolts you out of a deep sleep at 6:30 AM. Just as the remnants of a dream start to slip away from your consciousness, you notice another one of those mild cramps. This doesn't feel anything like what you've seen in the movies when women are in labor, so you heave yourself out of bed and into the shower. You only have three more days at work before you go on parental leave, and you can't wait. You get out of the shower and, as you're getting dressed, you notice another crampy feeling. Given these are feelings you haven't yet experienced in pregnancy, it seems only right to let your doula know. You text her at 7 AM, letting her know that you've been having crampy feelings on and off since 3:30, but that they are mild and don't seem very frequent or regular (you could sleep through them!), so you're going to work. She texts back with an excited emoji, and asks you to drink some water, put your feet up, and time the cramps for the next hour, before you go to work. She wants to figure out if they are Braxton Hicks or labor. You do that, but there are only two, and so you get up and drive into work.

Your day at work feels long, but it is made more interesting by some random crampy feelings that elicit excitement every time you have one. While you let your best friend at work know that you're feeling crampy and it might be labor, no one else knows and you feel like you're hiding the most thrilling secret.

After work, you go home and reheat some soup from the night before. After dinner, you plop down on the sofa with your feet up, turn the TV on to the most ridiculous reality show that you love, and revel in what you realize could be some of your last childless moments. As you watch, you notice that the crampy feelings are getting a bit closer together. You text your doula and she asks you to time them again for an hour. You grab your phone and open the timer contraction app. You've heard that 511 number floated around a lot, so you Google it to remember what it means. Right. You don't need your provider until the cramps are 5 minutes apart and 1 minute long for 1 hour. And there comes another cramp. You start the timer when you first begin feeling it, and then hit the stop button when your stomach softens again.

After an hour, you've found that your cramps are 7-10 minutes apart and they are about 30 seconds long. You text your doula with the information and she tells you that you're likely in early labor and should alert your midwife. So, you call your midwife and let her know what's happening. She listens to you talk through one of your contractions, and then tells you to nourish yourself, hydrate, and rest. She agrees that this seems like early labor, but this stage can last hours, sometimes even days.

You go on like that all evening, eat a delicious dinner, and then lie down around 9 PM to watch a show. You ask your partner to choose the most boring show they can think of because you really want to be able to fall asleep. If this is labor, you need your energy! You drift off to the sounds of the TV, only to awaken at 10:30 PM to a cramp that is stronger and that wraps around from your lower back to your front. Okay, this one feels pretty real. You get out of bed, so as not to wake your partner, and go into the bathroom, where you stare at yourself in the mirror, eyes wide open, marveling at the fact that this is probably it! You'll know your baby soon! And then, another cramp starts, and while it isn't in any way painful, it is a bit more intense than your average period cramp. You're timing these now and decide to go downstairs to do some cleaning to keep your mind off of things. After an hour, you find that they have settled into a predictable pattern, 6 minutes apart and about 45 seconds long. You go wake up your partner, who looks back at you with those same wide eyes you had an hour ago, and ask that they come support you. You also text your doula, letting her know your status. You don't feel like you need her just yet, but she lets you know that her bag is packed and she's ready to jump in the car the second you need her. It feels so good to know that she will be there to support you.

Likely the beginning of active labor

You and your partner spend the next hour downstairs, your partner dozing on and off, while the two of you watch your favorite comedy. You keep timing, and over the next two hours, your cramping becomes more intense and you find yourself needing to get up, lean against the wall, and sway your hips as your abdomen tightens and the cramp spreads from your lower back and around your belly. While the sensation is new to you, it isn't bad, and honestly, you are able to convince yourself that it's your uterus giving you and your baby a reassuring hug. Around 2 AM, you find that your contractions are getting more intense and are now 4 minutes apart and about a minute long. You go to the bathroom because you feel like you need to poop, and notice some bloody mucus-like discharge. You've heard of something called bloody show. Maybe this is that? You text your doula and ask for her to come now and then get on the phone with your midwife, just as another contraction starts. As she hears you lightly moaning through the pressure, you hear her calmly say, "I'm on my way. Be there in 20 minutes."

Within 20 minutes, your doula, midwife, and midwife assistant have all arrived. You've never been more grateful to see anyone in your life. Your contractions are coming quicker. Your partner says every three minutes now, and you're now starting to moan through each of them. Sometimes it feels good to walk, other times it feels good to be on a birth ball, and other times it feels best to be in the shower. But always, it feels good to have your partner apply pressure to your hips. Your midwife asks if she can check your dilation, and you decline. You'd *rather just go with what your body seems to intuitively know—how to birth your perfect baby. She does check you with a doppler though, and you hear your baby's reassuring heartbeat.*

You eat some yogurt, and keep hydrating. You don't know how long this will go on, but you want to be strong for your baby.

As time progresses, you lose track of it. You're so focused on going inward, on handling the intense pressure of the contractions, that time no longer seems real. The power of your uterus is remarkable. You knew it would be intense, but it seriously takes your breath away as each wave brings your baby closer to you. In between waves, you rest in silence. And during waves, you repeat the mantras that you practiced during pregnancy:

> *This is temporary.*
> *My body knows what it's doing.*
> *Each wave brings my baby closer to me.*

Transition

The surges are now so intense that you're moaning loudly (in low tones like your doula has taught you) and sometimes swearing a bit under your breath. They feel like they are coming one after another with no break. You look your partner in the eyes, grasping tightly to their arm, and emphatically tell them that you can't do this. You're done. When your midwife calmly tells you this means you're in transition and will meet your baby soon, you plead with her to make it stop. You tell her you're hot as you rip your shirt off, having completely lost all sense of modesty. Her calm energy is reassuring though, as she tells you that there are so many others going through this exact same feeling right now. She suggests that we call on all of their power, and together use it to bring new life into this world.

With that, you start to feel like you're going to poop again. You tell your midwife that you have to poop, and she says that your baby is getting closer. As you walk to the bathroom, an intense wave takes over. You lean into your partner to cope, and at the same time, feel your water burst all over the floor.

The pushing phase

You go sit on the toilet, dripping water, and feeling like you have to poop. But when no poop comes out, you realize that the downward pressure you feel is your baby. And you start to feel an intense need to push.

You're shuttled quickly off the toilet and back into your bedroom when an intense surge comes with the desire to push. You're working with your body to birth your baby. At this point, you've gotten down on your knees, with your upper body draped over your bed. Your midwife tells you that you should go ahead and push with each surge, as your instinct tells you to. And so you do. You don't know how many pushes, or for how long. You marvel at the strength you didn't know you had within you as each push gets your baby closer to you. With some pushes, you can feel your baby getting closer to you while you're pushing and then retreating back in when you stop, but you know that that's by design. Your baby and your body are working on stretching your birth canal so that you don't tear. You are determined at this point. If you've made it this far, you can do anything. And you do. Suddenly, just after the burning sensation of your baby's head almost makes you lose control, you feel their tiny body slip out of you–and now, you're sitting back, umbilical cord coming out of your vagina, with a beautiful baby attached and screaming on your chest. And you're crying. So much. You did it.

The golden hour and birthing your placenta

You spend the next 30 minutes marveling at this tiny creature who you already love with every cell in your body and thought in your soul, while your midwife pushes a bit on your now deflated belly. You barely even notice when you birth your placenta because your baby is nursing and it is the sweetest sensation you've ever felt in your life. What a miracle today is. The sun shines in the window, as it's now 6 AM, and you are so present in this moment that each ray feels distinct, golden, and magical. You are so grateful.

I've given you this picture of what birth has looked like for millennia and how it can unfold when medical interventions are not part of the picture. While the details of birth can vary from one woman to the next, and from one birth to the next (see my birth stories at the end of the book to see how that can look), overall, it is a physiological process that will result in a baby. When fear stops progress or when medical interventions are added to the equation, or both, labor can look very different. We will touch a bit on the impacts of such interventions throughout the book, and you can use this information to either make a decision or decide where you need to do more research. While this can be the only birth book you ever read, it can also be supplemented by advice from your doula or your childbirth education class, and it should definitely be integrated with advice from your provider.

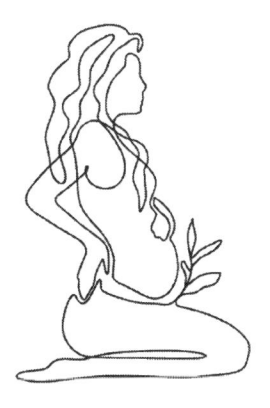

Conversation 5

Two pink lines—now what?

Whether you've been trying to conceive for years, or not trying to conceive at all, when you peed on a stick and got those two pink lines, your heart likely skipped a beat. You may have been in a state of disbelief. Perhaps there were tears. Perhaps, as was the case for me when I saw two surprise pink lines, you paced back and forth, exclaiming, "No f#%*ing way." Perhaps you were so excited that you couldn't help but squeal with delight. Maybe your heart started beating quickly, your eyes opened wide, and you felt terrified. Or did you feel a combination of many or all of these feelings at once? Whatever the immediate emotion upon learning that we are becoming parents, many of us are left not knowing what to do next. I'd like to take you through that now.

Choosing your birth place and your provider

Prenatal care is essential to the health of your baby. This means that one of the first things you should do after getting that positive test is to choose a provider (if you don't have one already). If you already have a provider, this is the time to ensure that they are aligned with your birth philosophy. If you don't already have one, this book will help you to form one. There are generally five different types of providers (plus doulas) and three different types of birthing locations. These are the most important decisions you'll make during your pregnancy and will likely determine what sort of birth experience you have. Let's get into the nitty gritty.

Types of providers

1. **Obstetric-gynecologists (OB-GYNs)** are trained as surgeons in traditional medical schools. Doctors are the most common birth attendants in the United States, attending 92% of hospital births.[54] They attend births in hospitals and often view pregnancy and birth as medical conditions. If you have a high risk pregnancy (e.g., you have placenta previa, pre-existing health conditions like auto-immune disorders or cancer, or develop pre-eclampsia), an OB-GYN is likely the person who is equipped to take you and your baby safely through pregnancy and

birth. OB-GYNs almost always attend births in a hospital and are the go-to if you need a cesarean. In my experience, OB-GYNs have a wide range of attitudes toward birth, but they have all been trained that birth is a medical event that is safest in a hospital. They are trained as surgeons, so surgery is a tool in their toolbox. OB-GYNs often utilize a variety of interventions, including cesarean sections, to "manage labor," rather than letting it unfold naturally. As surgeons, they are very comfortable intervening surgically to perform a cesarean. If you see an OB-GYN, they will likely be part of a larger practice that you will rotate through during your prenatal appointments and you will not be able to predict who will attend your birth.

2. **Family doctors,** also known as General Practitioners are medical doctors who have gone through medical school and then completed a three-year family medicine residency. Family doctors used to commonly attend births, especially in smaller, more rural areas, but OB-GYNs have taken their place in many communities.[55] Family doctors are not trained as surgeons, but they can and do sometimes perform cesareans.[56] Their views on birth are often somewhere between an OB-GYN and a midwife in that they likely view birth as a normal

part of life, but are trained to attend births inside the existing medical system, with all of the medical birth interventions at their fingertips. They usually attend births in hospitals. In more rural settings, a family doctor could be the person who provides prenatal care and who attends your birth, which offers continuity of care that is different from what you'll experience in a suburban or urban setting with an OB-GYN.

3. **Certified Nurse Midwives (CNMs)** are first trained as nurses in traditional nursing schools and then undergo a Master's degree in midwifery to become a CNM. They usually attend births in hospitals, but can also be found in birth centers and sometimes at home births. They attended 1 in 7.4 vaginal hospital births in 2018 in the United States.[54] CNMs are trained in low-risk, unmedicated, vaginal births. They often have more tricks up their sleeves to manage the intensity of birth without pharmaceuticals and usually are able to devote more time to building a relationship with you at your prenatal appointments. That said, many CNMs work in practices of multiple providers, so you may see a different CNM at each prenatal appointment and there is no way to ensure that your favorite CNM will be the one to attend your birth.

4. **Certified Professional Midwives (CPMs)** are not trained as doctors or nurses, but instead are focused primarily on pregnancy and birth as their specialties. Before attaining licensure, CPMs are required by the state (regulations vary) to complete educational programs in midwifery, to have attended a specified number of births, and to have provided prenatal care to a certain number of women. In some states, direct-entry midwives, who have learned primarily through apprenticeships with experienced midwives, are able to pass a certification exam to attain their CPM license. CPMs attend births at out-of-hospital birth centers and at the client's home. In states that require CPM licensure (36 as of 2021),[57] they are the most frequent attendant at home births. Like CPMs, they are well-versed in how birth unfolds physiologically without pharmaceutical intervention and are often particularly attuned to optimizing the mind-body connection for an optimal birth experience. Many CPMs will perform your prenatal appointments in the comfort of your home and they will almost always be the person to attend your birth. If you are interested in seeing the same provider throughout your entire pregnancy, and then knowing that person will also attend your birth, a CPM is your best option. Similar to CNMs, CPMs will be able to assist you

in doing the work to optimize your mind-body connection and have many non-pharmaceutical tricks up their sleeves to help you manage the intensity of birth.

5. **Direct-entry midwives (DEMs)** are found in the states that do not require CPM licensure. They have acquired their knowledge of pregnancy and birth primarily through apprenticeships and attend births at home or in an out-of-hospital birth center. Many DEMs are well-respected in their birth communities, but there is no regulation in place to ensure a high standard of care. This doesn't mean that a DEM can't be an amazing choice, but instead that you are solely responsible for ensuring that their experience and care philosophy match your expectations to ensure a safe birth. DEMs vary widely in the source of their knowledge and experience, but largely see birth as a natural physiological process. Similar to CNMs and CPMs, DEMs can assist you in optimizing your mind-body connection and provide you with non-pharmaceutical tools to manage the intensity of birth.
6. **Doulas** are not trained as medical professionals and so can only attend birth with a trained birth professional (whether doctor or midwife). Doulas are trained to provide emotional support during

pregnancy and especially during birth. Many are certified by accrediting bodies like ProDoula or DONA, but some are not. Research has shown shorter labors, fewer cesareans, fewer instrument-assisted births, babies with higher Apgar scores (indicating healthier newborns), and higher birth satisfaction for women who are supported continuously throughout labor.[58–60] Your doula will be your support throughout your pregnancy and will be there with you continuously throughout your birth. They will empower you to prepare, plan, and advocate for the birth experience you want, and will emotionally and physically support you throughout your birth with a variety of tools designed to create the best possible birth experience.

Given this, before we go further, I'd like to suggest that no matter what sort of provider you choose, you should also hire a doula. You'll want to choose a doula who you feel comfortable with, whose energy you really like, and someone who is confident enough to help you learn how to advocate for yourself. That's right, your doula shouldn't be advocating for you. Instead, they should be empowering you with the information you need to be able to advocate for yourself.

Now that you know about the types of providers and where they attend births, let's dive a bit deeper into what birth looks like in these different birthing locations.

Birthing locations

Hospitals are still the most common place to give birth in the United States. Let me walk you through an average hospital birth experience, recognizing that it can vary widely depending on (1) your ability and desire to advocate for yourself and (2) on the hospital and provider you choose. When you arrive at the hospital, you will go straight to the labor and delivery ward, where you'll be put into a small room in triage and hooked up to a monitor. The monitor is a belt that goes around your belly and monitors both your contractions and your baby's heartbeat. You may be asked to put on a hospital gown at this time. (Although it's up to you whether you want to do that.) In some cases, you will be asked to temporarily leave your doula and/or support person in the waiting room. Ask about this at your hospital tour if you're choosing a hospital birth. The nurse will be seeking to assess the frequency and duration of your contractions in order to determine whether you are in labor. They will also likely place an IV in your arm at this time and start you on a saline drip to ensure that you are hydrated. In most cases, the nurse will perform a cervical exam to assess how dilated you are. Once it is determined that you are in labor (i.e., you are sufficiently dilated and your contractions are regular), you will be transferred to a labor and delivery room. Your support person can usually rejoin you at this time.

The labor and delivery room will have a hospital bed and usually a chair. Sometimes, you'll be provided with a birth ball, a peanut ball, or other tools that will make labor more comfortable. You'll likely have access to a shower and, in some cases, a bathtub. If you are in a midwife-staffed birth center within a hospital, these comfort tools are more likely to be there. If not, you'll have to ask for them. You will now spend the duration of your birth in this room. If you choose an unmedicated birth, you may be able to walk the halls.

A nurse will likely ask you how much pain you are experiencing and whether and when you'd like an epidural. It should be noted that the traditional hospital birth model of care sees birth as a painful and somewhat risky process, which is why you'll be offered pain relief and monitored continuously using electronic fetal monitoring throughout your birth. Being hooked up to an IV, an epidural, and a monitor can make it more difficult to move around and, in the case of the epidural specifically, will limit the number of positions that you can birth in. You will spend most of your birth alone with your birth support person (e.g., your partner and/or doula), but the nurse will check on you occasionally. The midwife or doctor will likely check in periodically but won't spend any significant amount of time with you until you are pushing.

The ambiance in a hospital room is hard to improve, but in many cases you can turn off the lights to try to create a calmer environment. You can also bring in printed birth affirmations to decorate the walls, battery-powered candles to create better lighting, and your own music (bring a speaker in case they don't have one). Your doula will be particularly helpful in creating the right ambiance and keeping the room quiet for you.

If you choose to have an IV, an epidural, and continuous fetal monitoring, you will likely spend most of your labor in bed. When it comes time to birth your baby, the doctor or midwife will come in and tell you when and how to push. You are likely to push on your back, although many providers are now more open to a variety of more physiological birthing positions (which may be limited if you have an epidural). If you have an epidural, you won't be able to feel when or how to push in the same way that you would if you birthed unmedicated.

It is possible that you will have residents, nurses, the anesthesiologist, and the doctor or midwife in the delivery room as you push. You should also know that, in most cases, you will not be able to ensure that your normal provider is the one to attend your birth. If you get lucky your provider may be the provider on call. But in many cases, you may not have ever met the provider who attends your birth.

Once your baby is born, assuming no complications, baby will usually be put immediately on your chest (although this isn't always the case). If the provider is worried about your baby's health, they will take baby to an incubator across the room. In many hospitals now, the provider will do all necessary checks and medical care while your baby is laying on you. The provider will assign Apgar scores at 1 and 5 minutes after birth. The Apgar score assesses skin color, heart rate, reflexes, muscle tone, and respiration. You will likely be encouraged to nurse during this time, as you wait to birth your placenta. You can call on the nurses for assistance with breastfeeding if they aren't already helping. Most hospitals also have lactation consultants available if you have any problems. Many providers will administer Pitocin to assist with the birth of the placenta and to reduce the risk of hemorrhage. They will also likely pull a bit on the umbilical cord to guide the placenta out. Once a bit of time has passed (this varies by hospital and provider, but is ideally after the baby nurses), the baby will be weighed and measured. Antibiotic eye ointment (to prevent an eye infection that could develop if the mother has chlamydia or gonorrhea) will be placed in their eyes and they will be given a shot of vitamin K (to help with blood clotting). Once everything is cleaned up, people will leave the room and you will be left to nurse and get to know your child.

A home birth is exactly what it sounds like. Your midwife comes to your home and stays with you throughout your entire labor and delivery. This means that you have full control over the ambiance of your birth, and you will know the people who occupy your labor land. For the two home births I had, I ensured that our floors were spotless. (There was NO WAY I was walking on crumbs while having a baby!) The candles were lit and Indian classical music played quietly. You could do the opposite and throw crumbs all over the floor while you listen to death metal. It's up to you. The environment is yours. When birthing at home, the midwife will come to you once you're a bit further along in your labor. She will come to your home equipped with all of the tools needed to ensure a safe birth experience for you and your baby. She will monitor you intermittently, usually using a handheld doppler to check the baby's heart rate. You will eat, drink, and move as you choose.

For my second child, I labored in my bathtub but birthed her on hands and knees in the very room in which she was conceived. For my third child, I joyfully vacuumed and made my kids dinner in early labor. Later on, I labored in a birthing tub and birthed him in the water with my sister, kids, husband, and midwives in attendance, also in the very room in which he was conceived. If you are curious, you can read my full birth stories at the end of this book.

Your midwife is trained in normal, physiological birth. She will be watching you for signs that things aren't quite right, and will be prepared to transfer you to the hospital if she senses that you need the additional support. After the birth, baby will be placed immediately on your chest (you might catch baby yourself if you choose to!) and then you will nurse your baby in your own time, with the midwife's help. As in the hospital, midwives will record Apgar scores at this time. Most midwives allow your placenta to be birthed naturally, which usually happens within an hour. After the baby and placenta are born, and you have spent a substantial amount of time nursing and bonding while your midwives clean up the house, they will perform all necessary health checks on your baby, including weighing them, measuring them, and checking their reflexes. Eye ointment and vitamin K are options you can choose, but not all midwives automatically offer them. They will also examine your placenta to ensure that it emerged in whole. Many midwives will then offer an herbal bath for you and baby (which is one of the best parts of home birth!). Finally, once you're both in your own comfortable bed, clean and nursing, and the house looks like nothing ever happened, they'll leave you to sleep and revel in your new family together.

Birth centers are somewhere in between a hospital and your home. There are two types of birth centers: hospital birth centers and out-of-hospital- birth centers. In both cases, the environment is designed to be more comfortable than a hospital, more like your home. Rather than a hospital bed, you'll likely have access to a regular full or queen sized bed. You will likely be able to at least labor in a tub, and in some cases give birth there as well. You'll be monitored intermittently rather than continuously. In most cases, you won't be hooked up to an IV and you won't be offered an epidural. Many birth centers do not have the ability to offer you these interventions. In the case of a hospital birth center, you can experience many of the benefits of home birth (within the confines of any hospital policies) while still being close to a neonatal intensive care unit or an operating room should you require a cesarean.

How do I choose?

Some of you already know what sort of provider you prefer and where you'd like to give birth. If that is you, awesome. Go forth and prosper. (But make sure you have the information you need to make sure you actually are choosing the type of provider you think you're choosing.) For the rest of you, ask yourself the following questions. (See the figure below to remember what the acronyms mean.)

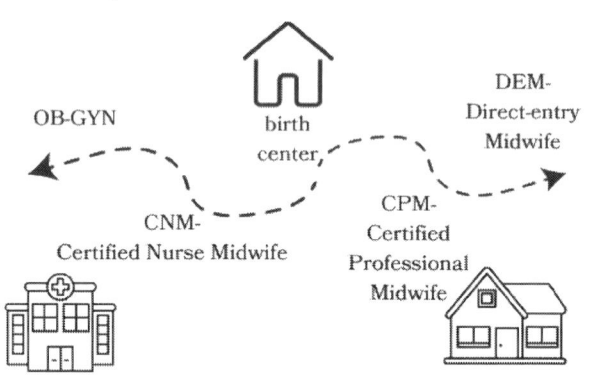

OB-GYN

birth center

DEM- Direct-entry Midwife

CNM- Certified Nurse Midwife

CPM- Certified Professional Midwife

1. Do I want to have time to ask lots of questions during my prenatal appointments?
   - If yes: consider a midwife (CPM, CNM, or DEM)
   - If no: consider any option (CPM, CNM, DEM, or OB-GYN)
2. Do I want my provider to be trained to help me succeed in having an unmedicated vaginal birth?
   - If yes: consider a midwife (CPM, CNM, or DEM)
   - If no: consider any option (CPM, CNM, DEM, or OB-GYN)
3. Do I want access to pharmaceutical pain relief?
   - If yes: consider a hospital (OB-GYN)
   - If no: consider a home birth or birth center (CNM, CPM, or DEM)
   - If maybe: consider a hospital or hospital birth center, or a home birth with the potential to transfer
4. Will I feel most comfortable if I am able to move freely during birth without being hooked up to anything?
   - If yes: consider a home birth or birth center (CPM, CNM, or DEM)
   - If no: consider a hospital birth (OB-GYN)
   - If maybe: talk to your provider about whether this is possible in your chosen location

5. Will I feel safest when I am in the same building as a NICU (neonatal intensive care unit) and/or an operating room, in case of an emergency?

> If yes: consider a hospital or a hospital birth center (**OB-GYN** or **CNM**)
> If no: consider a home birth or out-of-hospital birth center (**CPM** or **DEM**)
> If maybe: consider a home birth or out-of-hospital birth center that is in close proximity to a hospital AND talk to your midwife to understand under what conditions she would transfer you to the hospital. Make sure you are comfortable with her plan and confident in her abilities.

6. Will I feel safest if I know the people who will be there when I birth my baby?
   - If yes: consider a home birth (**CPM** or **DEM**)
   - If no: consider a hospital or birth center (**OB-GYN** or **CNM**)
   - If maybe: talk to your provider about the likelihood of knowing the person who attends your birth

7. Am I high risk? Do I have a pre-existing health condition that puts me at a higher risk of birth complications?
   - If yes: consider a hospital birth attended by an **OB-GYN**

- If no: consider any option (CPM, CNM, DEM, or OB-GYN)
8. Would I like to have my other children (or maybe my dog?) with me?
    - If yes: consider a home birth or potentially a birth center (CPM or DEM)
    - If no: consider any option (CPM, CNM, DEM, or OB-GYN)

Now that you've gone through these questions, go ahead and tally how many votes you have for a hospital, birth center, and home birth. Do the same for providers. Use that information and the information in the coming conversations to guide your decision. And know that even if you choose one provider, after you ask them the following questions, you might decide to switch. If you're able to ask your provider these questions during your interview or first visit, that will allow you to feel more confident in your choice from the beginning of your relationship together. This is a relationship. Don't forget that. They are there to provide advice and help you to safely meet your baby. You are putting a lot in their hands, so you want to make sure you feel confident in their abilities and that you trust them. While it's never too late to switch providers or birth locations, it's easier to do so early in your journey to parenthood.

Questions to ask your provider

How far along will you be comfortable with me going before you want to induce?

We have been taught that pregnancy lasts nine months, right? Guess what, it doesn't. We now think of pregnancy as lasting 40 weeks (10 months!), but that actually includes the 2 weeks in between the first day of your last menstrual period and the date that you ovulate and conceive. Before we talk about asking your provider how long they are comfortable with you cooking that baby in your belly, I want you to throw away the idea of a due date. Due dates based on your last menstrual period are inaccurate, and while those based on early ultrasounds are a bit better, one study found that only 25% of women gave birth by 39 weeks and 5 days and only 50% by 40 weeks and 5 days.[61,62] With that, I want you to think of a birth month as the due date plus or minus two weeks. So, if you are due on September 1, then your birth month will be approximately August 15-September 14.

Research has shown that 4 in 10 women indicated that their provider attempted to induce labor, with over a third of those inductions performed because the provider was concerned about the women being overdue or the baby being too big.[63] While there are valid medical reasons to induce labor (e.g., placental abnormalities, poor infant growth, preeclampsia),[64] doctors often recommend inductions simply because a woman is nearing her due date or because the baby is too big (you'll learn more about this when you get to Conversation 6.) While many inductions are successful and the most recent research no longer suggests that inductions increase the risk of cesarean when compared to waiting for birth to happen naturally,[65] women who are induced are often less satisfied with their births.[66–68] I don't know about you, but it's hard for me to feel empowered when I'm dissatisfied. Of course, if we compared rates of cesareans in women who were induced (18.6%)[65] versus those who planned home births (<6%),[69,70] the risk of cesarean would be substantially higher for women who were induced. A review of the scientific literature examining women's experiences of being induced found that women did not feel like they were included in the decision to induce. Those whose inductions ended in cesarean were disappointed. They didn't know why an induction was booked by their provider. They weren't educated on the process of induction. They felt unsupported during labor. And, they felt a loss of control over the birth process, with some even citing feeling like they were treated as a number rather than a person.[68]

Many providers will allow you to wait until 41 or 42 weeks (depending on your birth preferences and risk factors) to induce labor.[71] After 41 weeks, the risk of stillbirth increases ever so slightly, so that may feel like a real reason to empower yourself with the choice to induce labor. However, many providers feel comfortable with you waiting until 42 weeks if you have no other risk factors for stillbirth. If you are full term, nearing your due date, and you'd like to encourage labor naturally, you can go for long walks, eat dates, have sex, get acupuncture, use evening primrose oil, and engage in nipple stimulation. For anything else, talk to your provider. Once you are full-term, you can talk to your provider about sweeping your membranes (through a vaginal exam that can separate your bag of waters from your cervix) to induce labor in a painless and drug-free way.

I want to stress here that **there are valid medical reasons to be induced**. Ask your provider what those are so that you are prepared if you develop a complication that requires induction during your pregnancy. Be empowered now to make the best decision when the time comes! The most important part of all of this is to talk to your provider and ensure that you're comfortable with what they are recommending and their philosophy on labor induction. If you get to the point of talking about needing an induction, make sure you understand why an induction is being recommended and what the experience will look like. Find a provider you trust so that you are able to make an informed decision, even if that decision is to induce. You have hired them, they did not hire you. Make sure you're aligned now rather than scrambling to find a new provider when you're so big that it's hard to roll over in bed!

How long will you allow me to be in labor?

OB-GYNs were historically trained to believe that labor should progress according to something called Friedman's Curve.[72] Friedman was a doctor who observed 500 birthing women at a hospital in New York City and then graphed their average dilation curves. Some of these patients delivered with forceps, some had cesareans, and 98% were sedated either mildly, moderately, or deeply during labor. All that said, these data (which were based on highly medicalized births) dictate that the average first-time mother should progress to 10 cm in 14 hours. Friedman's Curve has been used by hospitals around the world to assess whether a woman is experiencing what the medical establishment calls "failure to progress." I like to call this "failure to use evidence." The good news is that the American Congress of Obstetricians and Gynecologists (ACOG—the authority on medicalized birth) created new guidelines in 2014 that are based instead on updated information and no longer recognize "failure to progress" as an evidence-based term.[73] These new guidelines recognize that active labor doesn't begin until 6 cm (instead of the 4 cm dictated by Friedman) and allow for longer normal labor durations.[73,74] They now have clear guidelines in place that are based on evidence, but unfortunately, old habits die hard. Even after these new guidelines were released, doctors continued to recommend and perform cesareans based on the outdated guidelines created by Friedman in

1955.[75] Ask your provider what their guidelines are for labor progression, how those change if you are induced, how those change if your water has broken, and then ensure that you feel comfortable with their answer. You deserve to be cared for by someone who has not only your and your baby's safety at heart, but is using evidence-based practice and is committed to helping you find your power through birth. The last thing you want is to be disempowered and unnecessarily put on Pitocin (which creates stronger and more painful contractions)[76] or to have a cesarean when there is no real reason to do so.

Can I labor without an IV?

If you are interested in having an unmedicated birth, you will need to be able to move around to manage the pressure of your powerful uterine muscles. Lying in bed will make it hard to manage. If this is your goal and you are choosing a hospital birth, ask your provider if you will be able to forgo the IV. One good alternative if they insist on an IV is to have them place a heparin or saline lock instead. This will allow them a quick port to your vein in the unlikely event of an emergency, without needing to be hooked up to an IV cart unable to easily move about.

Can I labor without continuous fetal monitoring?

If you are laboring in a hospital, it is likely that they will put two belts around your belly that continuously monitor your contractions and baby's heart rate. While they do this to increase their ability to monitor your baby without being continuously in the room with you, this will limit your mobility (which ironically can increase the likelihood of your baby's heart rate indicating distress).[77] Some hospitals have mobile, waterproof, continuous electronic fetal monitoring units that allow you to move around. Regardless of whether you are mobile or not, continuous monitoring may increase the likelihood of the provider using some mechanical method (e.g., forceps or a vacuum) to pull your baby out and the likelihood of a cesarean.[78–80] Unfortunately, this risk is not balanced by higher rates of healthier babies. Continuous electronic fetal monitoring does not reduce the risk of cerebral palsy; increase Apgar scores (indicating healthier babies); or reduce the risk of admission to the neonatal intensive care unit, brain damage, or death.[80]

If you labor at home or in a birth center, your baby's heart rate is more likely to be monitored intermittently using a hand-held doppler. While this type of monitoring is safe and less likely to lead to additional interventions, it is not common in hospital settings where nurses have to attend to multiple births at the same time. This is despite ACOG's admission that continuous monitoring has not improved outcomes for women with low-risk pregnancies. While they recommend that care providers should be trained to use a handheld Doppler device to allow freedom of movement,[81] these recommendations are rarely followed. It should be noted that even if you are low-risk, choosing an epidural puts you into the high-risk group with regard to the need for continuous fetal monitoring.[76] Ask your provider what method of monitoring they use, and if you'd prefer to be more mobile with a lower risk of additional interventions, you might request handheld doppler monitoring.

What is your philosophy on birthing positions?

The vast majority of births in 21st century America occur with the woman lying on her back, legs held up in the air by either stirrups or nurses with a doctor sitting at her vagina waiting to catch the baby. While this position can be necessary if you have an epidural that results in limited sensation in your legs, it is often pushed by providers to the detriment of people wanting an unmedicated birth. Doctors continue to ask women to birth on their backs despite loads of evidence suggesting that other birthing positions open the pelvis wider and result in better maternal comfort, quicker deliveries, and fewer complications.[82–84] Indeed, even ACOG noted that birthing on your back can have negative effects when they said "the traditional supine position during labor has known adverse effects such as supine hypotension and more frequent fetal heart rate decelerations."[81] This means that you might experience low blood pressure from lying on your back while baby's heart rate might slow down. Many people intuitively choose upright birthing positions likely because they know that it makes sense to allow gravity to work with them. When their intuition is challenged by providers who want them to lie on their backs for their own convenience, they are made to feel small and powerless.

Prior to the 1700s in Europe, it was more common for women to birth in ways that instinctively felt right, which meant that they were often upright when birthing their babies. During the 1700s, births began to be attended by men instead of female midwives and those men wanted to more easily access the baby emerging (and make it easier to use forceps to hurry the delivery).[85]

Many doctors and some CNMs will recommend that you birth on your back, especially if you have an epidural. Most CPMs and direct-entry midwives will let you decide what feels right. For example, I birthed my oldest child on my side, my second child on hands and knees with my upper body supported on my bed, and my third child on my knees with my upper body draped over the edge of the birth pool. I don't have the notes for my first two births, but for my third birth, I got out of the birthing pool to pee at 8:49 PM, then got back in and started pushing at 8:58 PM. My son was born at 9:05 PM. That means I pushed for only 7 minutes! Because I birthed unmedicated, I instinctively knew what position felt best to me.

Can you imagine a squirrel being told by another squirrel that she needs to lay on her back to birth her babies? The idea is somewhat ridiculous. What I want for you is the ability to choose when the time comes. You might decide that birthing on your back is right for you, and I want that for you if it is YOUR CHOICE. But I don't want you to be in a situation where you want to birth in an upright position or on your side and are forced, because of hospital or provider protocol or opinion, to birth on your back. Research shows that women who choose their birthing position have a shorter second stage of labor (i.e., they push for a shorter time).[83] You know your body and baby better than anyone. Trust yourself.

Will I be allowed to eat in labor?

Birth is seriously hard work. Mine were short in duration, but I needed nourishment to power through. For me, I drank chocolate coconut water and ate vegan yogurt. Chocolate coconut water brings back beautiful memories of birth and will forever be a comforting drink for me. While the World Health Organization and the American College of Nurse Midwives recommend that women be allowed to eat during labor if they desire, ACOG still advises that women in labor should not eat, but can drink clear liquids.[81] It seems doctors are afraid women will aspirate if they end up having a cesarean (they are more preoccupied with preparing for something unlikely rather than nourishing women to support the more likely, healthy, complication-free, unmedicated birth). If you tend on the hungry side, find out what your birth location and provider allow. Advocate for yourself. And worst-case scenario, ensure that you are well-nourished when you arrive at the hospital.

How many people will be in the delivery room with me?

Are you the sort of person who feels overwhelmed at a party? When you're there, do you seek out the one person you know and talk to them the entire night, from the sidelines? If this describes you, then this question is particularly important. But even if it doesn't describe you, please pay attention. For some of us, we can go so deep into labor land that we don't notice who is around. For example, with my first I ripped my clothes off in the birth center and honestly, it would not have mattered if the president of the United States was there. But during my second birth, because it was slower, I noticed who was in the room with me.

Let's revisit the idea that fear slows down labor.[86] Fear can even cause dilation to reverse. While this isn't well-accepted among physicians, midwives call this cervical recoil or reversal.[87,88] If you don't know the people who are in the room with you, there's a world where having them there might slow down your labor. This is particularly true if you feel uncomfortable or have any negative emotions about anyone in the room. Many women report their labor slowing down when they arrive at the hospital or when someone walks in the room who makes them feel uncomfortable. During your average hospital birth, there will be multiple people, most of them strangers to you, in the room. If that's a possibility for you, I recommend you ask your provider to limit the people to those they consider essential.

Do you recommend I hire a doula?

Most providers now recognize that doulas make their job easier by improving maternal comfort, reducing the risk of cesarean, reducing the rate of interventions, and improving neonatal outcomes.[89,90] With that, they usually welcome doulas. However, that isn't always the case. One study found that half of doctors have negative attitudes toward doula care.[91] Many doulas find themselves needing to defer to physicians in ways that do not indicate relationships of mutuality and respect, but are required in order to be able to find their place in the hospital delivery room where the medical provider holds the power. If you choose to hire a doula, and the research suggests that you absolutely should, make sure you talk to your provider ahead of time to ensure that you aren't creating tension in your birthing room. If your provider isn't enthusiastic about a doula, it might be best to find a different provider.

What is your episiotomy rate?

An episiotomy is an incision on the perineum, the skin and muscle between your vagina and anus. Episiotomies have historically been performed to reduce the risk of perineal tears. Ironic, right? Episiotomy rates vary widely around the world, from 4% in Denmark to 12% in the United States to 100% in Taiwan.[92] While episiotomies plus forceps can be an alternative to cesarean in select cases where a baby is truly stuck (e.g., in cases of shoulder dystocia that can't be corrected by maternal position), episiotomies are not without risk and are no longer recommended except in very specific circumstances.[93,94] Please ask your provider what their episiotomy rate is and look up the episiotomy rate of the hospital you're birthing at. (The Leapfrog Group has ratings posted online.)[95] Both should be less than 5%. While this is a tool that can save your baby's life, it should only be done in cases where the baby's life is truly at risk.

What is your cesarean rate?

A cesarean section (a.k.a., c-section) is a surgery that is performed when a doctor has ascertained that either the baby's or mother's life are at risk during birth. One in 3 women in the United States have their baby via cesarean.[96] In Brazil, that number is 1 in 2. Compare

that to Norway, where less than 1 in 5 women have their

Figure 2: Percentage of births that end in cesarean

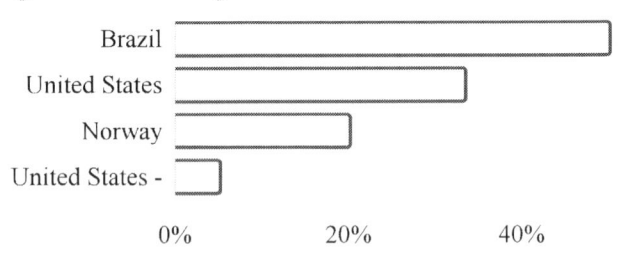

Brazil	~45%
United States	~30%
Norway	~17%
United States - home birth	~5%

babies via cesarean. In even starker contrast, only 1 in 20 women who planned a home birth in the United States ended up with a cesarean (see figure 2).[97] The most commonly cited reasons by physicians for performing cesareans are "failure to progress" (debunked in Conversation 5), fetal distress, fetal presentation, twin birth, and prior cesarean.[98] If we consider a cesarean rate of about 5% to be ideal (based on the home birth data), then that means that 83% of American women who had cesareans probably did not need them.

I want to be clear that I am not judging anyone who feels empowered by choosing a cesarean. But I am concerned about the person who feels pressured into a cesarean by medical providers who may be in a hurry to go home for the weekend,[99] may be avoiding a lawsuit,[100] or may be themselves afraid of birth. We talked earlier about fear being the driving force behind unnecessary interventions during birth. Remember, I am talking about fear in both the birthing person and the provider. Talk to your provider to ensure that they feel confident in their ability to help you have the birth you so desire, and that they see cesarean as a last resort to save your life. Remember, cesareans are major surgeries that carry a risk of maternal death almost four times higher than a vaginal delivery.[73] Birth is a natural physiological process that is safer than surgery. As I said earlier, there is a time for cesarean, but that time is far less often than our current medical system thinks.

For a hospital birth, ideal cesarean rates should fall under 20%.[101] But in my opinion, it is even better if you can get closer to the 5% cesarean rate seen in planned home births.[97]

How many unmedicated births that ended in vaginal delivery have you attended?

Many OB-GYNs have never attended an unmedicated birth. If your birth vision includes moving around, pushing in whatever way you see fit and maybe birthing in the water, you should ensure that your provider is supportive of your choice. Many providers will say they are supportive (and they likely are), but please also ensure that they have sufficient experience to demonstrate that they can support you in creating the ideal conditions to allow an unmedicated vaginal birth to unfold (if that is what you desire). If they have only attended a handful of unmedicated births (which is likely in a hospital setting), that might be a signal to dig deeper. Ask them more questions about how they envision supporting you. If they genuinely seem supportive, please trust your intuition. Working with a doula can also help to ensure that your birth wishes are honored in a hospital setting.

What is your favorite part of attending an unmedicated birth?

This question is particularly revealing. I have an answer. When I have attended unmedicated births, my favorite part is feeling the power emanating from the mother as she rides the waves of birth. If your provider can't answer this question, they likely haven't attended many unmedicated births.

Can I do delayed cord clamping?

When your baby is born, they will still be attached to you, and to the placenta until you deliver it, via their umbilical cord. Most of us, having been influenced by the media, imagine our partner cutting the cord right after the baby is born. But recent research demonstrates considerable benefit to the baby if you wait until blood stops pulsing through the cord. ACOG recommends delaying cord clamping by up to one minute, citing benefits to your baby of "improved transitional circulation, better establishment of red blood cell volume, decreased need for blood transfusion, and lower incidence of necrotizing enterocolitis and intraventricular hemorrhage."[102] You or your partner can still cut the cord if you so desire. At the very least, you want to make sure your provider is on board with waiting a minute to cut the cord. The American College of Nurse-Midwives goes further in recommending you wait 5 minutes.[103] Ensure your provider is on board with this most recent evidence.

For a home birth, why and when would you decide to transfer to a hospital?

If you choose a home birth, it is essential that your midwife know the early signs of impending complications that could require a hospital transfer. You'll want to ask them which hospital they will transfer to (ideally within 20 minutes of your house), and if they have a relationship with the physicians at that hospital. (Ideally they do. But in some states physicians have been so hostile towards home birth that it becomes difficult to build those relationships.) Common reasons to transfer to the hospital include a labor that truly isn't progressing, fetal distress, postpartum hemorrhage, and respiratory problems in the infant.[104] Ask your midwife what they are looking for, at what point they will transfer, and how often they've had to transfer in the past. A good, experienced midwife will feel confident and safe in bringing you and your baby through a home birth, but won't be afraid to transfer if a real medical need arises (or if you decide you want to transfer).

Printable List of Questions For Your Provider (or copy this page)

1. How far along will you be comfortable with me going before you want to induce?
2. How long will you allow me to be in labor?
3. Can I labor without an IV?
4. Can I labor without continuous fetal monitoring?
5. What is your philosophy on birthing positions?
6. Will I be allowed to eat in labor?
7. How many people will be in the delivery room with me?
8. Do you recommend I hire a doula?
9. What is your episiotomy rate?
10. What is your cesarean rate?
11. How many unmedicated births that ended in vaginal delivery have you attended?
12. What is your favorite part of attending an unmedicated birth?
13. Can I do delayed cord clamping?
14. For a home birth, why and when would you decide to transfer to a hospital?

Trust your intuition

When you're having these discussions, I want you to trust your intuition. If you feel that your provider is dismissing your questions, making you feel stupid, or getting defensive, they are likely not the right person for you. Trust your gut on this. The worst thing to do here is to ignore your intuition and find yourself in the most vulnerable position of your life, with a human literally emerging through your vagina, with someone who doesn't make you feel powerful. Remember, one of your goals (beyond having a happy, healthy baby) is to use this experience to transform yourself. Don't discount that. You matter. Your provider should make you feel like you matter.

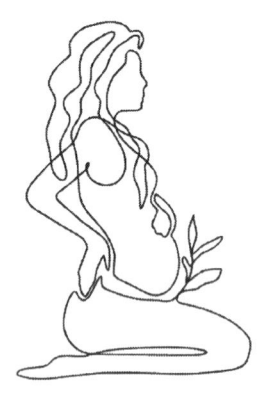

Conversation 6

What are your greatest fears surrounding birth?

We know that fear impacts the perception of pain, and hence our experience of childbirth, so let's talk about your fears. Here, knowledge is power. I want to disrupt any beliefs that have been created by the sensational view of birth seen in the media,[105] or by the risk-focused view of birth perpetuated by a Western medical system driven by profits and hence, the risk of being sued.[106] Fear and power don't mix well. Honestly, they are like oil and water. As part of finding your power, we need to unearth and disarm your fears. Let's replace them with visions of birth driven by love, knowledge, and power. I believe that all suffering on earth has fear as its root cause and birth is no different. Let's prepare you for an awakened birth.

Fear #1: Can my baby fit through my vagina?

Before experiencing birth, it may feel impossible to imagine how a human can fit your vagina. But remember, our bodies; including our birth canals, pelvises, and vaginas; have evolved to allow our babies to come into this world AND for us as parents to leave empowered so that we can keep passing on our genes (whether we choose to bring baby #2 or #3 into this world is another story). This means that your vagina is incredibly elastic and can stretch a great deal. Your baby works with you on this. Of course they do, because they're perfect already! The bones in your baby's head don't fuse together until years after birth so that their head can mold itself to fit through that 10 cm portal through your body as they join us on earth (and then their brain can grow larger throughout childhood).

We've all heard the story of a friend of a friend whose baby was too big to be born vaginally. Doctors for centuries have cited cephalopelvic disproportion, or having too small of a pelvis, as a reason why women cannot have their babies vaginally. Doctors and midwives have utilized a technique called pelvimetry to measure the size of a woman's pelvis. This technique is inaccurate,[107] which can result in unnecessary cesareans. While cephalopelvic disproportion is real, it is very rare, occurring in 0.4 percent of births.[108] If a woman is led to believe that her pelvis is too small to birth her baby, the fear she develops can make that her reality. Let me repeat that because it is important. If you are afraid that your birth canal is too small for your baby, you may end up creating that reality because the hormones associated with fear work counter to cervical dilation and effacement.[109] Indeed, research has shown that fear and anxiety are linked to increased epinephrine levels during labor, which are associated with a longer labor duration.[109] And as we noted earlier, those who have the most fear also experience the most pain.[52]

You can go ahead and put this fear aside. You are designed to birth your baby. Indeed, 99.6% of women have babies that can fit through their pelvis just fine![108] If you have a big baby, that's because your pelvis is large enough to birth a big baby. Keep repeating this to yourself: my baby fits easily through my pelvis because my body is designed to birth my own baby!

Fear #2: Will I tear?

An episiotomy is an incision made in your perineum, theoretically to allow your big baby to make their way out without resulting in a perineal tear (revisit fear #1). With recent research demonstrating that episiotomies actually contribute to rather than prevent perineal trauma, many doctors and midwives in the United States have stopped doing episiotomies.[26,110] If an episiotomy sounds terrifying to you (it does to me), check your hospital's rates[95] (and ask your provider how often they perform episiotomies). You can always choose a different provider, even late in the game. This is your body, your baby, and your birth. Take your power and own it.

While tearing is harder to prevent, there are things you can do to reduce your risk. The factors most likely to contribute to whether or not you tear include your choice of provider and birth location, how many babies you've had (first-time mothers are more likely to tear), bigger babies, family history of tearing, and interventions.[111] Many women swear by perineal massage during pregnancy as a way to reduce tearing. This involves massaging your perineum with oil (see Mongan's *Hypnobirthing* book for details).[112] Many midwives apply warm compresses during pushing and recommend laboring in the water. Regardless of whether you tear or not, the good news is that when a human is exiting your vagina, you aren't going to be focused on tearing. After the fact, if you do tear, your provider will give you a local anesthetic before stitching you up. I highly recommend you follow up with a pelvic floor therapist after your baby is born to ensure that you avoid long-term complications of tearing like pain and incontinence.

While no one likes the idea of any skin tearing, remind yourself that your body is meant to do this, and designed to heal. Think back to the last time you cut your finger. I always marvel at the magic of how our bodies just create new skin. Your perineum will do this too. Your body was made for this.

Fear #3: What if I don't make it to the hospital in time?

Precipitous labor, defined as labor that lasts only three hours from the beginning of regular contractions is incredibly rare, occurring in about 2% of women.[113] This means that your chances of having a baby in the car are slim to none.

I was in that 2%. My first birth lasted two hours, start to finish. It was precipitous. I was watching a movie on the couch (*The Twilight Saga: Breaking Dawn–Part 1*) around 10 pm, and just as the woman's stomach was cut open to free her body of the vampire baby that was sapping all of her energy, my water broke. No joke. Short story even shorter, my contractions started up quickly two minutes apart. When we arrived at the hospital a bit after 11, I anxiously awaited my husband as he parked the car. I sat in the lobby on one hip because I could *feel* a baby coming out of my vagina. Once I got to triage, the nurse attempted to check my dilation but instead exclaimed, "That's the baby's head!" Felix was born soon after, at 12:14 AM, just a few minutes after the midwife made it to my room.

Google's definition of a "precipitous action" is "an action done suddenly and without careful consideration." I will say, Felix's birth felt sudden and without careful consideration. It took all of my patience to hold on for what felt like an unexpected roller coaster ride. But I did hold on, and it was beautiful. I truly believe I wouldn't have had that amazing birth experience had I not prepared physically and emotionally.

When I was pregnant with baby #2, my main fear was whether I would make it to the hospital in time. When I expressed this fear to my midwife, she told me that I was a great candidate for home birth. My first pregnancy and birth were healthy, routine, and without complication. I was in my early thirties and in good health. And given that births often get faster with each additional child, there was a good chance that if I chose a hospital birth I might have the baby in the car.

All that said, if you are one of the somewhat lucky few who finds themselves plummeting through a precipitous birth, know that the vast majority of fast births are free of complications and end up with a (somewhat impatient) baby in your arms. Your birth is quick because you and your baby are ready for the ride, so why not put the top down and enjoy the wind in your hair?

Fear #4: How long will labor last?

This brings us to the next question, how long will you get to experience the roller coaster that is birth? The answer to this question is highly variable. I'll give you some statistics, but before we dive in, I want you to rethink time. Most of us are brought up believing that time is a fixed concept. We always want more time because we think our lives are dictated by time. But I want you to think of the last time you waited in line for your new driver's license at the DMV. One hour can feel like 12. And how about the last time you spent with your best friend, laughing? Three hours can feel like 10 minutes. Time is bendable. And when you are in labor, time no longer matters. But, in case you don't believe me, I'll answer your question.

The most recent research on duration of labor finds that it can take upwards of eight hours to go from 2 cm to 10 cm dilation (plus an hour or so for pushing).[114] On average, it takes a first time mom 6 hours to go from 4 cm to 10 cm. While you might hope to be average, know that averages come from a dataset of women who birthed for a wide range of labor durations. You could be at either end or anywhere in between. Some people have their babies precipitously in just a couple of hours, like I did with my first. Others can be in labor for days. What I want you to know though, is that if you are in labor for days, that does not mean that you'll be having intense surges two minutes apart for three days. Usually, longer births have a significant period of build up with irregular surges first that eventually space themselves evenly and then increase in frequency and intensity over time. I have not personally experienced long labors. But, I know that there are many women who have been empowered to let their body work with their baby to birth on their own timeline. They have used those longer labors to create even more moments of magic as they awaited the arrival of their babies earthside. It's all in how you see it.

While we're on the topics of fear and labor duration, we should revisit what I believe to be the most likely reason your labor will stall–and that is fear. A significant body of research proves that women who go into birth with fear have longer labors.[86,115,116] This makes intuitive sense. A woman awaiting the birth of her baby is in the most vulnerable position she will ever be in. Not only does she need to protect her baby as soon as they are born, but she has to protect herself at a time when she is not fully present in the world and is not in any place to defend herself physically. This is why mammals go into hiding to birth their babies. Safety. We need to feel safe in order for our bodies to birth our babies. Let me share a very basic, but very real, example.

When I was pregnant with my second child, I spent much of the afternoon having contractions that were seven minutes apart. I felt sure that I was in early labor. I picked my 20-month old son up from the babysitter after work. He had not taken his nap that day and so he fell asleep on the couch. I made dinner calmly, reveling in the quiet while my uterus continued to contract. After dinner, my son woke up from his very late nap and proceeded to spend the next 20 minutes or so screaming and crying (as small children sometimes do if they fall asleep at the wrong time). And guess what? My contractions stopped completely. My body knew that it wasn't a good time for me to be able to fully devote myself to birthing my baby, so it stopped the birthing process. My contractions didn't pick up again until the next morning with my daughter being born that night. Our bodies know what they're doing. Remember when I talked about the mind-body connection? This is the mind-body connection in action. I've even heard of women who have reversed dilation when someone they don't like comes into their birthing room! Imagine how disappointed you'd be to think you were 7 cm only to now learn that your cervix had closed itself up to 4 cm!

Get rid of your fears and embrace the adventure of birth.

Fear #5: What if I poop while pushing?

Are you worried that you'll poop while you push your baby out? Yes? Okay. This is an easy fear to address. You very likely WILL poop. You're going to be using the same muscles that expel poop from your body to expel your baby from your body. It's part of the process. Many of us get lucky enough that we feel like we need to poop BEFORE we get to the pushing phase. (Pooping is actually a positive sign that baby is coming soon!) The reason this is a lucky poop is because then you'll have less poop inside of you when you push your baby out. All that said, every midwife, doula, nurse, and doctor who has ever attended a birth knows that poop is just part of the deal. They aren't worried about it, and once you're focused on meeting your baby, you won't be worried either. Everybody poops. No big deal.

Fear #6: What if I have to have a cesarean?

First of all, having a cesarean does not mean that you can't still be empowered by birth or that your baby will be damaged. In my opinion, a truly necessary cesarean is simply a reminder that Western medicine is an amazing tool to have when we need it. If a cesarean is medically necessary, then use your power to let the doctors help you to have your baby safely and do so with gratitude. Power doesn't mean doing everything by ourselves. Power also means knowing when to ask for help.

That said, there are ways to significantly reduce your chances of having a cesarean. The biggest predictor of the level of birth interventions that you will experience (i.e., induction, epidural, forceps, internal fetal monitoring, and cesarean) is the location in which you birth and the provider you choose (see Conversation 5). Each intervention increases the chances of future interventions.[26,76] If a woman is induced with Pitocin, she is more likely to have an epidural. She will also be required to have continuous fetal monitoring, which makes her more likely to have a cesarean. Each intervention can lead to more interventions, so the place least likely to have interventions (at home or in a natural birth center) is also the place where you are least likely to have a cesarean.

While a birth center or home birth may be the best choice for many, not everyone should have their baby at home or in a birth center. You need to birth in a place where you feel safest. If the idea of birthing your baby in your own bedroom, away from the technological advantages of Western medicine, sends you into full-on panic mode, then a home birth might not be best for you (although this might also be a sign that you have fears to work through). But regardless of where you choose to birth your baby, if you are hoping to avoid an unnecessary cesarean, you should do your research on the hospital you choose and the provider you choose. If you choose a CNM, you are less likely to end up with a cesarean than if you choose an OB-GYN with a high cesarean rate. You see, your power begins the moment you begin to make decisions about who you want in the room, and where that room should be. You are powerful now, even before you give birth. And if you can own that power now, the possibilities are endless for what you will do with the power you unearth during birth. Get ready to change the world!

Fear #7: What if I lose control?

Birth is the perfect time to relinquish control, learn to trust and surrender, and let your uterus do the work for you. When I was preparing for my first birth, I did ALL the research and trained as if I were running a marathon. I took a Hypnobirthing® class. I listened to meditations and birth affirmations every day. I did prenatal yoga. I practiced my birth breaths. I read all the books about birth. I exerted my control by preparing for birth, and I'd recommend you do the same. Ironically, it is only after taking control of your preparation for birth that you will be prepared to relinquish control. The second my water broke, that control that I had cultivated evaded my conscious mind. The months of planning that had prepared my subconscious were absolutely necessary because I was no longer in conscious control. I was forced to surrender while my subconscious took over. When I was pushing my son out, my husband asked if I wanted him to read the list of birth affirmations I had so carefully prepared. I yelled "No!" at him because I was no longer in control. Instead, I was able to trust that my body, my baby, and the Universe would all work together to bring my baby earthside. And being able to surrender to the waves of birth gave me a taste of the beauty available to me in life when I can surrender and trust that the Universe has my back. Having learned how to surrender during birth, now every time I do the prep work that allows me to then surrender my problems, no matter what they are, and trust that the Universe has my back, I enjoy my life more.

I know some of you are wondering what it actually looks like to surrender. The idea of surrender feels intensely uncomfortable. I want to emphasize that when I surrender, that doesn't mean I don't also do the things that are necessary to achieve the outcome I'm hoping for. I still do those things. For example, when I was worried that we wouldn't be able to pay my kids' tuition, I did my very best at work (which I'd do anyway) in the hopes that I'd get a raise and a promotion. (They go to the best school in the world and so this is an essential cost for us.) But I also actively surrendered the problem to the Universe. I did meditations during which I envisioned us paying tuition easily and then handed that vision over to the Universe. Surrender does not mean inaction. Surrender, to me, means trusting that the love that is the Universe is here to take care of me—and if I take right action, I can trust the Universe to use me for the highest good.

Fear #8: What if the pain is too much?

We're back to pain. I know. You thought we already covered this. But seriously, if you believe the pain will be too much, it will. You'll insist upon an epidural the second you get to the hospital. And that may be the best route for you. It isn't the birth experience I chose, but part of your power is in your choice and plenty of people choose that route.

If you believe, however, that this sensation is intense pressure that will allow you to feel the earth-shaking power that you hold within yourself, then birth will not be too much for you. If you release all of your fears ahead of time and choose a birth location and provider that makes you feel safe, held, and cared for, the sensations of birth will not be too much for you. If you are seeking to connect to the Earth and Mother Nature and your place as a living being in this Universe, you can do so by riding the waves of birth. Billions of people for hundreds of thousands of years have come through childbirth stronger and more powerful. You can too. In the last 500 years or so, through a move towards birthing in hospitals rather than at home and excluding women from the medical profession, we have seen the patriarchy steal power from women during birth.[117] We have been told that we aren't good enough or strong enough, that birth is not a natural process and that it needs to occur in a place overseen by men. Take your power back. This is your chance.

And honestly, there may be certain situations when an epidural is a tool to help you find your power in birth. I am not here to tell you that epidurals are all bad; they are a tool that can help you to find power if you find that your unique circumstances have resulted in intensity that is leaving you feeling disempowered. Trust your intuition.

Fear #9: What if I hemorrhage?

Postpartum hemorrhage refers to excessive bleeding from your uterus after your baby is born. It is rare, meaning that about 97% of births do not result in maternal hemorrhage.[118–120] In one study that looked at women who had planned home births, over 99% of births were uncomplicated by postpartum hemorrhage.[118] Issues with your placenta, in either this or a previous pregnancy, increase the risk. If you have a placental disorder (i.e., placenta previa, placenta accreta, placenta increta, or placenta percreta), talk to your provider to ensure that you are both doing everything possible to birth your baby safely. If you don't have a placental disorder, then you are likely in the 99% who will not hemorrhage. Rest assured that if you do, your provider will be well-equipped to treat this condition. If this is bringing up fear for you, talk to your provider ahead of time to ask how they've managed this in the past, and then journal this out every day until your fear has diminished.

Fear #10: What if I don't connect to my baby?

We have all seen the movies and heard the stories of the woman who births her baby, only to fall instantly in love, crying tears of joy while she stares into her newborn's eyes. What you probably haven't heard are the stories of the woman who desperately wants a baby, gets pregnant, goes through a long and arduous birth experience, and doesn't feel a rush of oxytocin when she holds her baby for the first time. She may feel indifferent, and also then, confused. If everyone else falls in love instantly, why didn't she? And then she's left feeling like she's already failed at motherhood.

I'm here to tell you that parents (not just mothers) experience a wide range of emotions upon first meeting their baby, and that none of those emotions predicts what kind of parent they will be. Perhaps the mother just lived through a 36-hour labor. Exhaustion can definitely impact bonding at first. Or maybe they had an unexpected cesarean under general anesthesia that is altering their hormones and emotions. What I want you to know is that emotions are temporary. Every single one of them. The fact that you are even reading this book tells me that you are going to be an amazing parent who loves your baby, even if that feeling of love doesn't flood your emotions instantly. So if that's you, let it go. The love will grow. You might just need a nap first.

If you're particularly worried, you can increase your chances of bonding by building that relationship while you are pregnant.[121] Read to your baby. Talk to them. Sing to them. Play them your favorite music. Dance with them. It might feel silly at first, but they can hear you. There's no reason not to let them know how much you love them, even before they are born. I've created a meditation for you to bond with your baby (see Conversation 7). Do this meditation as often as you'd like and revel in the warm, fuzzy feelings.

Bonding can be particularly hard for those of us who have suffered from depression or who lacked strong attachments with our own parents. If this is you, please talk to your therapist while you are pregnant (this applies to a co-parent too) about how to get into the healthiest psychological space possible for your baby. Untreated depression during the first trimester of pregnancy can lead to postpartum depression.[122] Your baby needs the best version of you, and while none of us are perfect parents, just knowing that you're trying to work on yourself will demonstrate your love towards your child in ways they'll never forget.

If you find yourself feeling particularly sad or if you are having difficulty bonding with your baby in the early weeks, please talk to your provider and get help. Postpartum depression is common, affecting upwards of 1 in 5 women.[123,124] While your provider and your pediatrician should screen you for postpartum depression at your routine visits, if you are feeling unusually sad, anxious, overwhelmed, or depressed, please use your power and let your provider know. Postpartum depression is not your fault, and it is treatable. Your provider will have a depression screening tool that they can use to assess how you are doing. And if you aren't depressed, but are feeling anxious, please ask for the postpartum anxiety screening tool. Postpartum anxiety is even more common than postpartum depression, but often goes undiagnosed.[125] You and your baby deserve to enjoy this time together. It only happens once and it's fleeting, so please take care of your mental health. Remember, we all need to put on our own oxygen masks before we can help others.

Fear #11: What if I'm not a good parent?

Becoming a parent was and still is the most transformative experience of my life. Disclaimer: I don't like to fail at things. I wouldn't call myself a perfectionist, but I prefer to do things well. And parenting is the most important thing I do that I refuse to fail at. My first few years as a parent were tough. The transition away from considering only my own needs to also considering the needs of two tiny, demanding humans was not easy. I fought it every step of the way. While pregnancy and birth empowered me, the incessant screams of toddlers disempowered me. When they threw tantrums, I was taken back to childhood myself, to a time when I also didn't have control. And so I threw tantrums right back at them. I yelled at my toddlers. Yep. I'm writing a book on empowering yourself through birth, but I am not a perfect parent and I definitely wasn't a great parent when my babies were tiny. I am going to give you three pieces of advice that were game changers for me as a parent. I discovered all of these pieces of advice after my third child was born, during a time when I was forced to surrender. Fletcher was born with an airway disorder called laryngomalacia. This meant that for the first months of his life my sole purpose was to keep him alive. I sat upright at night holding him in just the right position so he could breathe. I stared at oxygen monitors that were attached to his tiny toes while he slept. During the day, I wore him in a carrier and, whenever he would look up at me with panic in his eyes because he was struggling to breathe, I took him outside and walked him because being in nature would calm him down. I knew exactly what my purpose was during that time. It was to be the very best parent I could be. And being so very present allowed me to grow.

Here are the three pieces of advice I'd like to offer you, as you begin on your journey as a parent.

1

Get to know your ego, and then tell your ego to f#%* off. It's the voice in our head that we can observe, the voice that tells us we aren't good enough or that things are not as they should be. For me, Eckhart Tolle was essential in my journey of self-discovery. Read his book, *A New Earth*.[126] Meditate. Recognize that your thoughts are not you. You are the beauty and love that observes your thoughts.

2

Nurture your child as THEY are, not as you want them to be. Dr. Shefali Tsabary's work was instrumental in my understanding that each of my children is a unique being and that their tantrums, their "misbehavior," are simply cries for help. Read *The Awakened Family* by Shefali Tsabary.[127] It changed my life and the lives of my children.

3

Truly hear your children. When my youngest was a toddler, I listened to a talk by Thich Nhat Hanh during which he described a practice called "deep listening." I believe he was talking about how to create real connection and love between people. I so wish I had gotten this piece of advice when my older two were babies, but alas, everything happens for a reason and I probably would not have been able to take it in and apply it then. He told me that when someone is expressing their upset to me, whether it be sorrow or grief or anger or frustration, that I should look them deeply in the eyes and calmly say, "I hear you." And then just be there with them. Don't solve their problem. Don't offer advice. Just hear them and be there with them as they experience suffering. While Thich Nhat Hanh recommended this for adults, it was a game changer for me as a parent and for my children. I want them to know that emotions are not their enemy, that all feelings will pass, and that they are there as a tool for us in life. But when my older two kids threw tantrums, I resisted. I desperately wanted those tantrums to end. And because of that resistance, not only did their tantrums last hours at times, but they learned not to trust their own emotions. I was teaching them not to trust themselves. For this, I am deeply sorry. But after the advice from Thich Nhat Hanh, I was able to apply this technique to my youngest from the time he was a toddler. When he wanted a different colored cup, or to go to the park at an inopportune time, or to play with a toy that his sister had, he expressed those desires the way any 2, 3, or 4-year old would, with tears and whining and sometimes screaming. But when he did that, I got down at his level, looked him in the eye, and calmly and with compassion said, "I hear you, Fletcher. It's really hard when you can't have what you want. I'm here with you." I'm still doing this now, as he turns five. And guess what, almost every single time I do this, he takes in a few deep breaths and lets the emotion go. Seriously. It's magical. I've tried this with other preschoolers, and with my older kids, and sometimes even with other adults and my colleagues. We each just want to be heard, and heard with compassion. You can do this for your child from the time they're a tiny baby just wanting to be held by you. Please take this piece of advice and apply it across your life, even to yourself. I wish I had always known this about humans.

✲

Now that we've talked through your fears, let's get into the nitty gritty of preparing yourself to be awakened and empowered by birth.

III

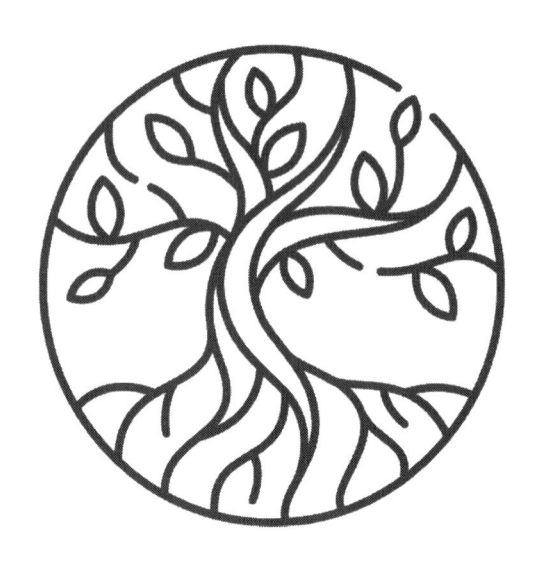

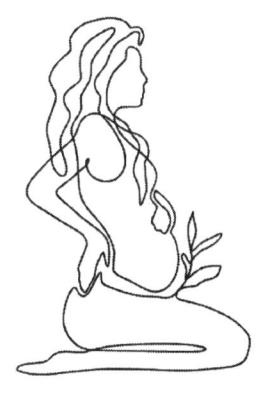

Conversation 7

Tools of empowerment

As I have mentioned a couple times already, you should be preparing like you're running a marathon so that you can then surrender and allow your power to take you through birth to get to the point where you have a baby in your arms. How else can you unearth your power? This next conversation will first give you the tools you need to dissolve your fears and then provide you with pregnancy and birth tools that will leave you so well prepared that when that first wave hits, you are ready to surrender. Let's create a birth experience that gives your baby the best start as a human and gives you the best start as a parent. While some of these tools will only be used during birth, some should be learned and practiced during pregnancy to allow them to have the most positive impact on your experience.

Tools to transform fear into power

Fear can slow down your birth. It can make birth more painful. It can put you at higher risk of developing complications. Fear will take your power away and prevent you from being awakened by birth. Look back on the fears in our last conversation and think about which you really identified with. If there are any that don't ring true to you, forget about them. They aren't your fears to hold. For those that did create a stir in your consciousness, let me give you some tools that you can use to remove these fears from your subconscious. The most impactful tool you have to find your power is to uncover and work through these fears.

1

Let your friends know that you are only interested in taking in positive birth stories right now. Your subconscious is like a sponge, and as you go about squeezing the fear out of it, you don't want to drop it into a bucket full of more fear. If someone starts to tell you their own horror story, here's what you say: *"Thank you so much for wanting to share. Right now, I'm doing the hard work of reversing the fears I have surrounding birth and I'd love your help with this. You can help me by saving your birth story until after I have my baby."*

2

Instead, listen to positive birth stories. *The Birth Hour* podcast is a great place to hear from others who have gone through birth and come out stronger.

3

Watch as many unmedicated birth videos as you can, and in each, notice the woman's power and focus on the fact that she ends up with a healthy baby in the end. That could be you. After each video, I want you to close your eyes and visualize your upcoming birth. Notice how it feels to have intensely powerful muscles that bring your baby close to you. Imagine that you feel like a goddess, because you are. You are literally a portal for people to enter this world. And then, imagine what it feels like to hold your baby after working so hard to bring them earthside. The joy is palpable. Feel it and enjoy it now. You can enjoy that joy every day by just closing your eyes and using your imagination. Our thoughts create our reality, and even if you don't fully believe that, it feels really good to just allow yourself to feel that joy anyway.

4

Read *Breaking the Habit of Being Yourself* by Joe Dispenza. He talks about changing your subconscious beliefs, and provides you with tools and meditations to do so. Per Dr. Dispenza, every time you notice any birth fear popping up in your day, say "CHANGE!", either out loud or in your head. Doing Dr. Dispenza's meditations with your perfect birth in mind, and literally feeling how you will feel when that perfect birth experience occurs, will help you to release any fears that are holding you back (and that could be keeping your cervix hostage when you are in labor).

5

Listen to birth affirmations (see Conversation 7) and "Rainbow Relaxation" by Marie Mongan. Do this every evening as you fall asleep. Be amazed.

6

Watch animal birth videos on YouTube. Notice how they seem to be fine. Do you really think that humans are designed to suffer immensely during birth while the rest of the animal kingdom is calmly birthing their babies?

7

Do you have any other fears? As you read, keep a journal by your side and write them down and then explore them. Journal about any of your fears. Sometimes just writing something down is enough to get it out of your head. It can be therapeutic to write, stream-of-consciousness style, whatever thoughts come into your mind. I've found that if I just keep writing about my fears, they feel less scary when I'm done. If that isn't enough, talk to your doula about your fears. Talk to your provider. Talk to friends who have been empowered by birth. We all have fears, but most of them are not based in reality. If you find yourself hitting a wall with a fear surrounding birth, I want you to pull on the positive, loving energy of all the people who have birthed all of the billions of babies who have ever walked on the face of this earth. If birth were something to be feared, would so many have gotten through it? Journal about that.

Here are some journal prompts to help you process your fears:

- What is your fear? Is it rational or irrational?
- What will happen if your fear comes to fruition?
- How can you prepare so that your fear does not come to fruition?
- What could your birth look like if you didn't have this fear?
- If you were truly in your power, how would your birth experience unfold?
- Does it make you uncomfortable to be truly in your power?
- What benefit do you get from giving your power away?
- What benefit would you get if you stood in your power?

I want you to revisit these tools any time you're feeling fearful. It's possible that those fears will bubble up more as you get closer to the end of your pregnancy. If that happens, double down and devote time every day to using the tools I provided to help those fears dissolve.

Tools to use during pregnancy

In addition to working through your fears, you'll want to use the following tools to prepare yourself during pregnancy. Empower yourself with knowledge through a well-designed birth class. Change your outlook on birth through the use of daily affirmations. Bond with your baby through the bonding meditation. And exercise, because, isn't exercise always good for you?

A birth class

You have probably already been bombarded by the overwhelming catalog of birth classes available to you. Lamaze, Hypnobirthing®, Hypnobabies, your hospital birth class, the Bradley Method®, Birthing from Within, Mama Natural, Evidence Based Birth® Childbirth Class, Know Your Options Childbirth Course, and your doula's birth class (among others). Birth classes are generally not one-size-fits-all. I recommend you look into each and choose the one that feels right for you. If you are able, take your childbirth course with a live instructor so that you can ask questions.

I took Hypnobirthing® and found it to be transformational, playing a huge role in my birth. While I do think most people would benefit from taking Hypnobirthing®, I'm biased when I recommend it because I simply haven't taken the other birth classes. Hypnobirthing® focuses on removing the fear from birth, changing the way you talk about birth (e.g., waves instead of contractions), and utilizing self-hypnosis to deal with the intensity of birth. You'll listen to a nightly meditation called "Rainbow Relaxation" and will learn breathing techniques that will help you to breathe your baby out gently (rather than pushing). This course focuses on the idea that birth isn't painful. Honestly, I think this largely worked for me in helping to reframe birth and understand the sensations of birth as intense pressure rather than pain. My only criticism of Hypnobirthing® is that it didn't prepare me for how intense birth is. I had expected a super calm birth during which I would breathe my baby out, but instead I was hit with a freight train of a precipitous birth. That said, my midwife and nurses commented on how calm I was during my two hour birth, and noted that it must be because I had taken Hypnobirthing®. For my second and third births, I was able to combine my knowledge of the intensity of birth with the purposeful calm of hypnobirthing to find my power. With that, I always recommend Hypnobirthing® to anyone hoping to find their power in birth.

Birth affirmations

If you are alive in the 21st century, you've likely heard that you can change your life through the use of positive affirmations that will change your attitude and create the habits you want to create, while helping you to get rid of any habits that aren't serving you. While much of the self-development world utilizes these tools without citing the science behind their effectiveness, rest assured that there is science to back this practice. Self-affirmations have been shown to help people decrease stress, increase exercise, eat more fruits and vegetables, reduce negative thoughts, and do better in school.[128–132] Research shows that practicing self-affirmations actually increases certain neural pathways in the brain related to self-valuation.[133] While I believe wholeheartedly in the power of affirmation in creating an empowered birth, it's heartening to see that there is also research that supports the use of affirmations in reducing anxiety during birth.[134]

How do affirmations work? Your mind is divided into the conscious mind and the subconscious mind. Your conscious mind is responsible for the purposeful actions you take every day. It's the part of your mind that reads a recipe and turns that recipe into a delicious dinner for your family. Your subconscious mind holds the knowledge that allows you to run on autopilot. It knows how to ride a bike or drive a car, which is very helpful. But your subconscious mind is also the storage place for deep-seated beliefs about the nature of the world. It's the repository for all of those images of the beet-red woman screaming in labor and all of those memories of our parents, teachers, and friends telling us that we aren't good enough. While it can be relatively easy to learn new information to be used by the conscious mind, it's harder to change the beliefs stored in our subconscious. Harder, but not impossible.

You can change your subconscious mind through consistent repetition. After all, that's how all of those current beliefs came to be! Please read the list of affirmations below, slowly, thinking about how each one makes you feel. Do you feel truth in any of them? If you do, awesome! Are there any that feel completely false to you? Those are the ones that we need to work through, the ones that are related to your fears. For those that feel false, I want you to talk to your doula and journal about them. If you have a therapist or life coach, talk to them about them too. Truly interrogate *why* they feel false to you. At the same time, repeat these every morning and night, out loud, feeling into the truth of them. Let yourself feel the positive feelings associated with them as you say them. Record yourself saying them and then play the recording on repeat as you fall asleep at night or while you're cleaning the house. Write and rewrite these in your journal each day. Do any combination of the above! We want to reprogram your subconscious.

1. Just like every other mammal on earth, my body is designed to birth my baby.
2. My baby fits perfectly through my birth canal.

3. My uterine muscles are strong and gentle, designed to hug my baby as they peacefully enter this world.
4. I have the same power as all birthing people for all millennia.
5. I birth my baby easily with the power of all women/people as the driving force.
6. Each wave is temporary and brings my baby closer to me.
7. My baby feels my love as I bring my baby earthside.
8. I am grateful for the strength of my uterus.
9. I am grateful for each wave because it brings my baby closer to me.
10. I am curious about the sensations of birth.
11. I have dissolved all fear surrounding birth and replaced it with excitement, curiosity, and gratitude.
12. I am strong.
13. I go inward to a place of deep focus as I birth my baby.
14. My baby and I are connected and work together.
15. I design a safe, comfortable birth environment conducive to ultimate relaxation.
16. I am relaxed during birth.
17. From the strength of my uterus emerges my power to bring a new human earthside.
18. My muscles are loose and relaxed and my baby slides through easily.

If you think of new affirmations as you go, by all means, add them to the list. If you want to change the wording so that it sounds more like you, please do so. This is your birth, not mine. Own it!

As you get closer to your birth month, print out your favorite affirmations on cards and then have your support people place these in your birthing room. If you have been practicing them throughout your pregnancy, they will be even more powerful during your birth.

Bonding meditation

Find a quiet place to sit comfortably. You can record yourself saying this meditation, and then play it back to yourself. Leave a minute or so between each prompt so that you have time to truly connect with your baby. I recommend doing this meditation at least once a week, but you can do it every day if you wish.

Close your eyes and let the thoughts go from your mind. They will keep coming, and each time they do, just let them fade away like a leaf traveling away from you down a meandering stream.

Notice your breath as it comes into your nostrils. Notice the cool feeling of the air on your nostrils as your chest and belly rise.

And notice the warmth of the breath as you breathe out through your nostrils. This breath has gone through your lungs to nourish your baby. Your baby feels love with each breath you take.

Revel in the connection of your breath to your baby's well-being. As you breathe in, you send nourishment to your baby. As you breathe out, the love that you feel for your baby grows.

Now notice where your belly sits in space. This home for your baby is the perfect home. Through healthy eating, exercise, prenatal care, and love, you have created the ideal environment for your baby to grow. Your baby can feel your love as you engage in healthful practices that nourish them. With each breath, your belly rocks back and forth, soothing your baby. You are the perfect parent for this baby, and they are the perfect baby for you. Notice that rocking and feel the connection between you and your baby.

Each time you feel your baby stir, no matter what you are doing, notice the secret connection that the two of you share. Only you know what it feels like to have your baby move around in your womb. And only your baby knows what it feels like to be nourished and loved and to grow in the perfect environment of your womb. This is a special connection that only the two of you share. With each breath, that connection grows stronger.

Feel the intense love that your baby has for you. I want you to imagine your favorite color now and imagine yourself enveloping your baby in loving energy of that color. The intensity of that loving energy builds and builds each time you sit with your baby like this.

Place your hands on your belly and imagine love radiating out of your hands to hold your baby. Sit in this loving energy for as long as you desire.

Notice how you feel when you do the bonding meditation with your baby. Revel in those feelings. You can find moments throughout the day to bond with your baby. Rub your belly and tell your baby how wonderful they are! What a beautiful adventure you and your baby are on together.

Exercise

Stay active during your pregnancy. Most people can continue most activities that they engaged in pre-pregnancy throughout their pregnancy (but always check with your provider). If you were a runner, keep running. If you danced, keep dancing. If you did yoga, by all means keep doing yoga. You'll want to avoid activities that risk a fall or some other force to your belly. Don't wrestle or play tackle football!

Both research and anecdotal evidence show that women who exercise throughout their pregnancy have healthier pregnancies and easier births. Anecdotally, I want to share that I ran and did yoga throughout all three of my pregnancies, and I felt so powerful once I got to game day. Research supports the need for exercise to support a healthy pregnancy and a powerful birth. Studies show that exercise reduces the risk of pre-eclampsia[135] and gestational diabetes.[136,137] The results also pay off during birth. Women who practiced Pilates during pregnancy had less intense sensations during labor, shorter labors, pushed for less time, and were more satisfied with their births.[138] In short, they were more empowered. Another study found that women who did yoga during pregnancy were more likely to have a vaginal delivery instead of a cesarean, had shorter labors, were more comfortable during labor, and had fewer low birth weight babies.[139] Aerobic exercise during pregnancy leads to shorter labors, an increased ability to deal with the intensity of sensations during birth (and hence a reduced likelihood of using an epidural), and a reduced risk of having a very large baby.[140] If we combine these results with all of the research demonstrating that exercise makes people happier, it seems like a no-brainer. Stay active during your pregnancy!

Tools to use during birth

Water therapy

I was fascinated by the idea of a water birth from the moment I was pregnant with my first. But the stars didn't align until my third birth when I learned that birthing my baby into the water was magical. He didn't need to transition from the aquatic world of my uterus to the air-breathing world until I already had my hands on him, pulling him to my chest. I have to wonder if that transition was easier than if he went immediately from my uterus to the cold, foreign feeling air. Regardless of his experience, what I know for myself and what many others have attested to is the fact that water is calming during labor. Whether the feeling of water running down your back and belly, or the feeling of weightlessness on your body at a time when the pressure is already intense, water is healing.

If you choose not to have an epidural, many hospitals will allow you to labor in the shower or even a bath, but most won't let you birth in the water. Many birth centers do allow water births, and of course, you can always have a water birth at home. If this is a tool you'd like to have access to, especially if you're someone who enjoys water for relaxation when you aren't pregnant, please talk to your provider to ensure that you're able to have access to water. (You bath lovers, I'm talking to you!) Water birth has been shown to reduce the intensity of pain during labor, increase a feeling of control and empowerment,[141] and lead to more positive birth experiences,[142] all without any evidence that water birth is a risk to baby.[143,144] Even if you don't end up birthing your baby in the water, using water as a tool during labor can reduce anxiety, increase your satisfaction with your birthing experience, and reduce the sensation of pain.[145]

Massage and touch

You are going to be so excited to know that your partner and/or doula need to get on board with massaging you during labor! Research shows that women who are massaged during labor have less anxiety and pain, are less agitated and happier, and have shorter labors, shorter hospital stays and less postpartum depression.[146,147] They also have lower cortisol levels and, as a result, their babies were calmer during labor (as evidenced by less excessive fetal activity).[148] This one is relatively simple. Human touch is healing; use it during labor.

In addition to regular massage, light touch massage is recommended by Marie Mongan in her book on hypnobirthing. This involves someone lightly dragging the back of their fingertips up your back, moving away from the spine. This massage was essential to my success during my second birth.

Your doula will likely come prepared to use her hands to assist you during labor. As a doula myself, I've been at births where I alternated for 24 hours between hip squeezes and counterpressure to help my client surrender to each wave. I have seen the effectiveness of touch with my own eyes. I have massaged my clients in between surges and watched the anxiety and fear melt away. As a doula, I was so grateful to have these tools to take the edge off, which then allowed my clients to find their power.

Music

Have you ever been in a bad mood, driving in your car, when a song comes on that brings back positive memories, and your mood shifts? Music is extremely powerful at triggering our emotions. Use it to your benefit. Create a playlist with different types of music: upbeat, relaxing, powerful, light-hearted. And then you can choose what feels best for you while you birth your baby. It likely feels intuitive that music will help improve your labor experience. I probably don't even need to tell you this. But as you would expect, research demonstrates that music can reduce the perception of pain intensity during birth.[149-151]

Laughter

When you're in labor, most people wouldn't think to tell you jokes or suggest you watch Seinfeld reruns. But the old adage, "laughter is the best medicine," is based in reality. Laughter reduces the perception of pain in a variety of settings.[152,153] I've had clients listen to funny stories, and I've seen the effects on their perception of the sensations of labor. What makes you laugh the most? Is it a book or a stand-up routine? Whatever it is, bring it with you as a potential tool to use. I'm sure your baby will appreciate hearing your laughter as your uterus brings them earthside.

Moo like a cow and keep your mouth loose

This one is simple, but important. Once you get to the point when you feel the need to vocalize to deal with the sensations of birth, remember to moo like a cow. I got this piece of advice from one of Ina May Gaskin's genius books, and it works. You may find yourself wanting to shriek rather than groan. Don't do that. Shrieking will increase the intensity of sensation but a low moan will reduce the intensity of the sensations of birth. Ina May also says to keep the muscles in your mouth and neck loose, and in so doing, you will keep the muscles in your vagina and birth canal loose. You want to do whatever you can to release tension in your body. When you notice muscles tensing, relax them. Over and over and over.

Choice of words

You have likely noticed that I have used a variety of words to describe birth in this book. The words we choose can be critical to our empowerment during birth. If the word "contraction" elicits memories of screaming women, use the word "wave" instead (unless "waves" elicit fear in you). I don't advocate for any specific words because I find this to be highly individual. I, for example, had no problem using the word "contraction," but I wanted to avoid using the word "pain." I do suggest that you interrogate how different terms make you feel, and use those that benefit you. For example, research demonstrates that using the word "pain" actually creates a more painful experience.[154] For that reason, it may be wise to ask that no one asks you if you arc in pain during birth.

Here are potential alternatives to the common labor terms:

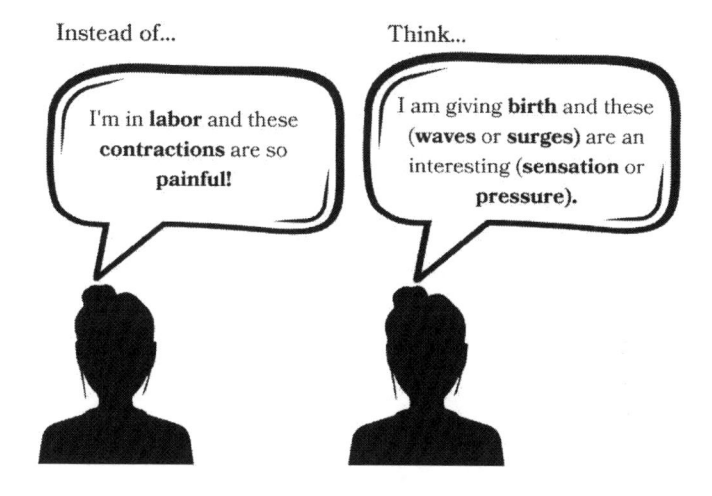

Instead of... — I'm in **labor** and these **contractions** are so **painful!**

Think... — I am giving **birth** and these (**waves** or **surges**) are an interesting (**sensation** or **pressure**).

Or maybe we should just go straight to your power.

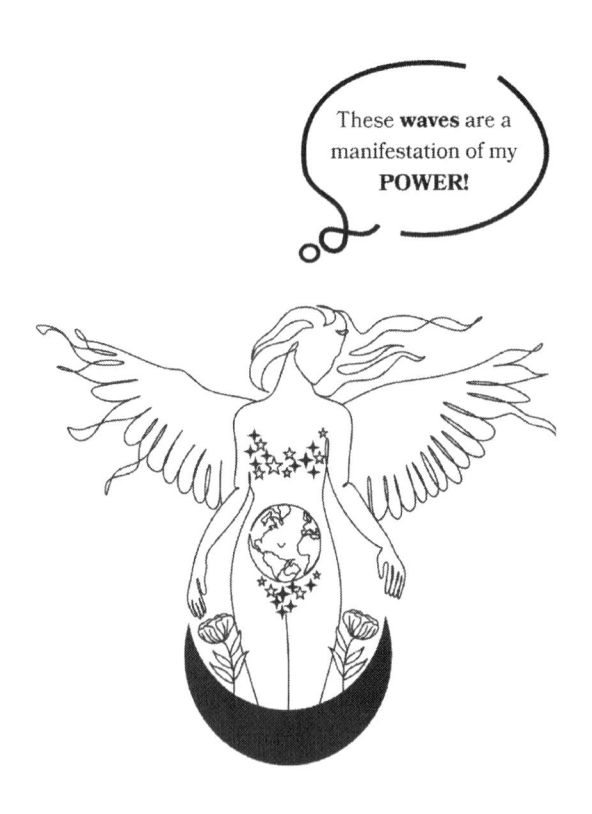

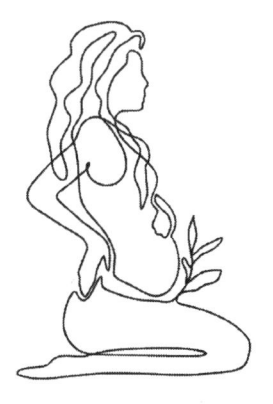

Conversation 8

Envision your perfect birth experience

Now that you have this information on birth, I want you to take the time now to envision your perfect birth experience. I've created a meditation for you to guide you through this process. You can record yourself saying this and then listen, or have someone read this to you. Please pause for a minute or so in between prompts to allow yourself to go fully inward.

Close your eyes. Notice the feeling of your hands. Are they tingling?

Now notice the feeling in your feet. Are they tingling?

Can you focus now on both your feet and your hands at the same time? Feel the tingle of energy in your cells.

Now focus on the feeling in your legs. Can you notice the heaviness of your legs and focus on the area around your legs? Feel the tingle.

Now do the same with your head and neck. Can you notice where your head and neck are in space? Feel the tingle as the atoms that make up your body and the electrons within those atoms vibrate.

Now feel the tingle of energy in your chest. Notice how your chest rises and falls with each breath, and feel the energy radiating out of your heart center. This is the energy of love. It is golden, like the nourishing energy of the sun that supports all life on Earth.

Now notice that energy of love radiating out of your heart center and direct it down to your uterus, the home for your baby. I want you to imagine the calming, loving energy glowing the gold of sunshine enveloping your baby in love and safety. Sit with your baby, feel the energy that their atoms are sharing with the atoms of your uterus and placenta, the amazing organ that you have created to nourish your baby as they grow inside of you. You are the perfect home for your baby, and they are the perfect baby for you.

Now imagine that your uterus has started contracting, your baby is telling you that they'd like to meet you soon. Where are you when you first notice that your baby is ready to meet you? Continue to envelop your baby in that golden energy as they work with your uterus to come through the portal of your body.

What are you doing now that you know you will soon meet your baby? Are you at home? In nature? At work going about your day? I want you to really feel the intense joy, excitement, and love that you will feel when you hold your baby. Truly feel that now.

The waves that are bringing your baby closer to you are getting stronger and closer together. It is time to call your provider. Where are you and what do they say to you? In your ideal birth scenario, how does this play out and what emotions do you feel? Imagine them now.

Now you are in the place where you will have your baby. What does the environment look like? Who is there with you? Is it quiet or noisy? Is it light or dark? What music is playing? Are there candles lit? Are the surroundings familiar or unfamiliar to you? Above all else, focus on how safe you feel in the environment that you have created. Notice the golden energy surrounding you and your baby in a field of love, safety, and joy. Sit and feel those emotions now.

Your uterus is sending waves through your body that are bringing your baby closer to you. Feel the strength and power that overtake everything you are at this moment. Stand in your power, knowing that you are creating the exact birth experience that your baby needs to thrive in this world. Sit with the feeling of calm and satisfaction that emerge with your power.

You can feel your baby low down in your pelvis now, entering the birth canal. You know that your body is designed to birth your baby. All fears and worries were released weeks ago, and now you are here, strong and powerful and ready to meet your baby. Go inward. Feel the calm concentration in that golden energy that every birthing person has drawn from since the beginning of time. That energy is here to support you through this.

Now that your baby is traveling through your birth canal, who is around you? Is anyone touching you? Supporting you? Are you in a bed, on the floor, or in water? What music is playing now? What is the lighting like? Who will be the first person to touch your baby? Imagine your ideal birth environment and feel the calm that comes over you as you realize that you are here and your baby is emerging.

Your baby is now in your arms. You look into each other's eyes. Feel the intense joy and love. You have drawn on your power to create the ideal environment for your baby to enter this world. Feel proud. Feel joyful. Feel satisfied. Sit in these feelings for as long as you'd like.

Now that you have envisioned your perfect birth, write down as many details as you can. You can use these details to guide you as you learn more and advocate for yourself and your baby. I'd encourage you to do this meditation weekly, or even daily, throughout your pregnancy. As you learn more, your vision might change, and that's okay. Part of this process is learning what you desire for you and your baby, and then surrendering once you are in labor, knowing that you have done everything you can to prepare.

Once you feel like you have your vision in place, you can begin to create a birth plan. Review your plan with your support people (e.g., partner or doula). Take this birth plan to your provider for their input and to make sure they are supportive of your wishes. And then take copies of this birth plan with you to wherever you decide to birth your baby.

Writing a birth plan

As you are envisioning your perfect birth, you will be preparing yourself to write a birth plan. The birth plan should address your preferences regarding the following topics. Please note that most of this applies to a hospital setting. If you choose to birth at home or in an out-of-hospital birth center, much of this will be your standard birth experience.

Throughout labor and birth:

- *Desire to have all interventions explained and to be permitted bodily autonomy (i.e., the right to choose):* This one may be the most important. You're reading this book because you're hoping to unearth your power through birthing your baby. No matter where you choose to birth, you'll want to talk to your provider ahead of time to let them know your plan and ensure they're on board with you finding your power and exercising your autonomy during birth. Put this at the top of your birth plan.
- *Ambiance of the room (e.g., lighting, music, essential oils, noise levels):* Remember, you are seeking to create an environment that makes you feel safe. Fear will slow down your labor, and you may need to focus inward

during birth. It is up to you to create that environment. If you are birthing in a hospital, you might want to bring twinkle lights, candles, your own music and a speaker, and an oil diffuser with oils to create that ambiance. You'll need to ask staff to keep the noise levels down if that's what you're hoping for.

- *Who you would like in the room:* If you want to ensure that your partner or birth support person stays with you at all times, say that. You'll only be allowed one support person if you end up having a cesarean. Otherwise, you can make your preferences known here regarding who can be in your room. If you want to keep it to essential staff (e.g., no students), make that known.

Early and active labor:

- *Use of epidural or other pain medications:* If you are planning an unmedicated birth, state that here and ask that the nurse does not ask you if you are in pain or if you'd like pain medications. You can use this section to ask to be given a hep/saline lock instead of an IV.
- *Use of Pitocin or other labor augmentation methods*: You can use this section to reiterate your desire for an unmedicated birth and that you be permitted to labor as long as is possible in accordance with hospital policies. Remember, you'll want to find this out ahead of time. Ask your provider how long and under what circumstances they'd require you to be

given Pitocin or other labor augmentation. Because Pitocin causes your uterus to contract differently, if they decide to put you on Pitocin, you will be required to be monitored continuously and will have less control over your own mobility.

* *Desires regarding mobility and type of fetal monitoring:* It will likely be easiest for you to be most fully in your power if you are able to move around as you prefer. In addition to reducing your ability to walk around and use water therapy (unless you have a waterproof mobile monitoring belt), as we talked about in Conversation 5, continuous electronic fetal monitoring also increases your risk of other interventions, including a cesarean. Additionally, being continuously monitored can take your provider's attention away from you as a person and instead place that attention on the monitor. If you are low-risk, you can ask to be intermittently monitored using a handheld doppler or, at the very least, to be intermittently monitored using a continuous monitor that you take on and off.
* *Alternative comfort management preferences (e.g., water therapy, doula support, birth ball, etc.):* If you are aiming for an unmedicated birth, you'll want to ensure that your birthing location permits you to use any comfort management tools that you are planning. List them here.
* *Desires regarding eating and drinking during labor:* See Conversation 5 for more on this. In short, many

hospitals will only allow clear fluids. If you tend on the hungry side (or even if you don't), check with your provider ahead of time and note in your birth plan if you'd like to be able to eat and drink. If you are hooked up to an IV, they will likely give you saline for hydration. You can choose to self-hydrate instead. I recommend coconut water.

- *Cervical checks:* I went through all of my labors with no cervical checks. It's what I preferred because I trusted that my body knew how to birth my baby. All the squirrels and giraffes and hippos I knew about knew how to birth their babies without cervical checks, so I thought I could too. And I did. If you're birthing in a hospital, your provider may not like it, but it is 100% your right to decide whether someone checks your cervix. Some women want cervical checks so that they know where they are at. If that's you, great. But just know that you can choose to decline.

- *Words to use during labor:* Look back to the end of Conversation 7 when we talked about word choice. If you're trying to convince yourself that the sensation you're feeling is powerful pressure, having your nurse ask you if you're in pain can ruin your plan. Let your providers know your word choices ahead of time. Make sure they're on board. And then put them in your birth plan.

During second stage (pushing):

- *Coached vs. spontaneous pushing:* Having birthed all three of my babies with midwives who were particularly hands-off in their approach, I was surprised during my journey to becoming a doula when another doula told me that I'd need to help coach my client on how to push. This seemed akin to me teaching my client how to poop. But alas, when pushing with an epidural, you might not be able to feel the sensations of pushing very well. You would likely be on your back in a position that isn't usually chosen intuitively during birth. Under these circumstances, you really might need that help. If you're planning an unmedicated birth, you can ask not to be coached and to just allow yourself to push spontaneously when you instinctively feel the desire. If you change your mind, you can always ask for help once you're pushing.
- *Birthing positions:* If you would like freedom in choosing your birthing position (which is admittedly harder if you choose an epidural), you should make note of that here.
- *Avoidance of episiotomy:* Given the association of episiotomy with perineal tears, it probably makes sense to state that you'd like to avoid an episiotomy unless medically necessary.
- *Support of perineum:* There is a wide range of practices thought to prevent perineal tears by supporting the

perineum during pushing. Some providers are completely hands off and don't touch your perineum while you are pushing. Others apply a warm compress. Still others apply lubricant in the hope that it will help the baby slip out more easily. And still others will put their fingers into your vagina while you are pushing to try to stretch your perineum. There isn't a lot of evidence in support of these practices, but there also isn't a lot of evidence to show that it's harmful. Talk to your provider ahead of time and make this decision based on what feels right to you.

Postpartum (after baby is born):

* *Place baby on chest immediately—skin-to-skin:* Most hospitals and almost all midwives will place baby on your chest immediately after they are born, assuming there are no complications. The benefits of skin-to-skin contact between baby and mother immediately after birth are immense and backed by loads of scientific evidence. This time, often called "the golden hour," allows baby to more easily transition into the world outside the womb (both physiologically and emotionally), with less crying. This special time also allows the mother to birth the placenta more quickly, bleed less after birth, and bond more easily with her infant, resulting in an easier time breastfeeding.[155–157]

- *Delayed cord clamping & who will cut the cord:* Remember from Conversation 5 that, in order to give your baby the healthiest start, ACOG recommends allowing the blood from the umbilical cord to pulse for at least a minute before cutting. Midwives often recommend five minutes or until it has stopped pulsing. Many hospitals will do this automatically, but not all, so you'll want to find out and perhaps put this in your birth plan.
- *Placenta delivery:* Many hospital providers will manage the birth of your placenta by giving you a shot of Pitocin to cause your uterus to contract and expel the placenta and will pull gently on the umbilical cord. This Pitocin can also reduce the risk of hemorrhage. Many midwives, especially in a home birth setting, will let your body deliver your placenta naturally. The evidence on which of these methods is better is mixed.[158] After doing more research on this, if you feel strongly either way, I recommend you talk with your provider.
- *What to do with the placenta:* If you'd like to take your placenta home, either as a keepsake (I planted a cherry tree over one of my placentas) or for placenta encapsulation (which many women swear helps with postpartum depression), make sure your provider knows. Many providers and hospitals will have protocols in place, including potential blood testing ahead of time, before they will let you take your placenta home. It's a good idea to state this in bold

in your birth plan. If you are planning to take your placenta in capsules as a supplement, talk to your doula ahead of time so that you are on the same page about how she will get the placenta from you.
- *Antibiotic eye ointment, vitamin K, vaccines, and first bath:* In the hospital, these are all administered within the first day of baby's life. Do your research so that you can advocate for the healthcare you'd like your baby to receive.
- *Feeding preferences:* It's a good idea to let your provider know, in your birth plan, what your plans are for feeding your baby. If you're planning on breastfeeding, I highly recommend that you join a La Leche League group while you are pregnant and read *The Womanly Art of Breastfeeding*. This was my breastfeeding bible and helped me to successfully and joyfully nurse all three of my babies for three years each. If you are planning on breastfeeding, you'll want to think about whether you are comfortable with pacifiers and with formula. There are differing views on whether early pacifiers or bottles interfere with breastfeeding. I didn't give any of my kids pacifiers, which meant that I had no way to stop them from screaming in the car as babies (you should know that babies love to scream in the car!), but also that I never had to wean them from a pacifier. How you feed your baby is entirely up to you, but make sure you are purposeful in your choice.

A basic sample birth plan for unmedicated birth

Birthing person: Judy Treehouse (she/her)
Partner's Name: Johnny Treehouse (he/him)
Doula's Name & Phone Number: Wanda Wiley (she/her), 555-1234
Due date: July 1, 2024

- I am planning a vaginal, unmedicated water birth and prefer not to be offered pain medications. **Please do not ask me if I am in pain.** Instead, you can ask me about the intensity of the pressure.
- Please **explain all interventions and get my approval before moving forward**. In the case of an emergency, my husband can speak for me.
- I would like my birthing room to be kept as **calm and quiet as possible,** with dim lighting and music of my choosing. I would like to keep non-essential people out of my birthing room.

During labor, I would like:

- as few cervical exams as possible
- to move about freely
- to be monitored intermittently with a handheld doppler
- to labor without an IV, if medically possible
- to eat and drink freely
- to labor in the birthing tub

During the pushing phase, I would like to:

- to be monitored intermittently with a handheld doppler
- to labor without an IV, if medically possible
- to eat and drink freely
- to labor in the birthing tub

During the pushing phase, I would like to:
- push spontaneously, without coaching, in the position of my choosing
- hands off perineal care (i.e., no compresses or massage)
- to birth in the birthing tub

After baby is born, I would like:
- to catch my own baby
- to delay cord clamping until after the cord has stopped pulsing
- to wait on any newborn care (eye ointment, weighing, Vitamin K) until after the "golden hour" of baby lying on my chest
- to deliver my placenta without manual assistance or Pitocin, unless I am hemorrhaging

An effective birth plan should be short (no more than two pages) and to the point. Most medical professionals are busy and honestly don't have time to read something long. Make it easy for them by focusing on the most important points.

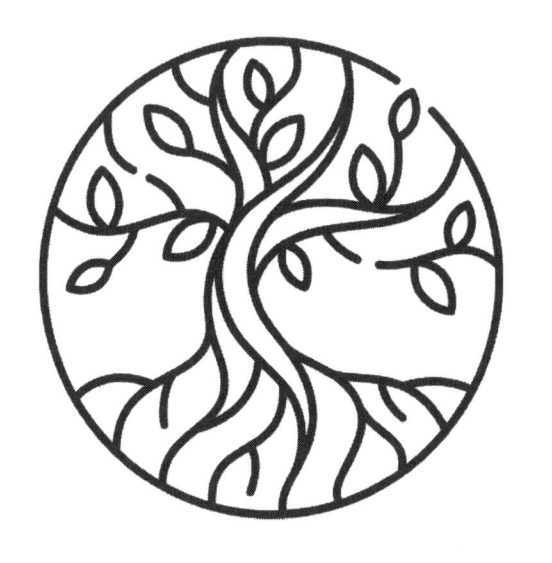

IV

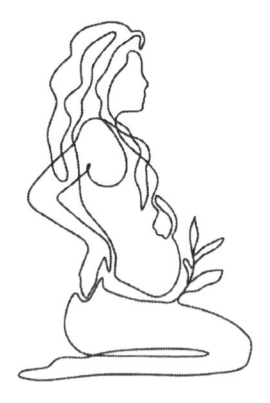

Conversation 9

My Birth Stories

This second to last conversation consists of my three birth stories. These were written when each of my babies was a newborn, so they are raw and real. I provide these not to say that this is how your births should go, but instead to let you know what drives me to write this book. Each of my births empowered me. Despite sometimes feeling like I wanted to quit in the middle of having my babies because it was physically the hardest thing I've ever experienced, I drew on my own power to persist, and when I succeeded, I knew that I could do anything. I am who I am today because I birthed my babies. I'm successful in my career because I birthed my babies. I've persisted through tough times because I birthed my babies. I'm an amazing parent because I birthed my babies. I'm a good wife because I birthed my babies. I can do anything I set my mind to because I have found my inner power through birthing my babies. I feel so fortunate to be able to share these stories with you.

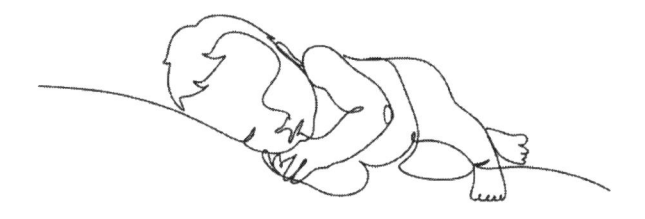

Felix Thomas
Born March 3, 2012 at 12:14 AM
Birth story written March 8, 2012

Last week, I woke up on Wednesday and Thursday nights feeling a little damp between my legs and thought maybe I was leaking amniotic fluid. Then Friday, we went to our normally scheduled midwife appointment. She checked my fluid and it turns out that I wasn't leaking. We spent the rest of Friday shopping for baby stuff. While we were at Target, I felt a little weak and like the baby was punching me down low, but I attributed my weakness to the fact that we hadn't yet eaten lunch. I even told Ryan, "I'm totally the kind of person who would be in labor all day but just blow it off like it was nothing." It turns out it wasn't nothing.

That night, we were watching a movie around 10 PM when all of a sudden I heard a pop and felt a small gush between my legs. I jumped up, saying that I thought my water might have broken, and ran to the bathroom. Once I got there, the water was still coming out, but after a few minutes, it stopped. Ryan and I went online and started

Googling to try to figure out the difference between my water breaking and peeing in my pants. While we were staring at the computer trying to figure it out, I started gushing again. At that point, we knew that I was in labor. I went and sat on the toilet and called the midwife answering service while Ryan rushed around the house trying to pack the things we needed for the hospital. (We still had 3.5 weeks to go and hadn't yet packed a bag.)

When I first spoke to the secretary for the answering service, she asked if I was having contractions, and I wasn't sure that I was yet. I felt a little pressure, but not an actual contraction. I hadn't started timing them, so I didn't have much to tell her. While I waited for the midwife on call to call me back, the contractions started coming pretty strongly. Once I realized that they were definitely contractions, I started timing them and found that they were two minutes apart (this was only about 20 minutes after my water broke!). I put a towel between my legs and rushed around with Ryan, trying to pack clothes to bring the baby home and clothes for myself to come home. The contractions got really strong really quickly, so I told Ryan that we had to leave. He packed the stuff in the car, and we took off.

By this point, the contractions were extremely strong. My reaction to them was funny. For one contraction, I'd use my hypnobirthing breathing, telling myself that it was only temporary and it was bringing my baby closer to me, and I'd be okay. But then the next one would come around so soon, and I'd start thinking, "What the f*!$ was I THINKING?!?!?! I can't do this!!!" Looking back on it now, it was really quite humorous. I'd expected that I would have time to get used to the surges, starting with ones that were far apart and building up to the strong ones that were close together. But, instead, I went from no contractions to really strong ones that were one on top of the other!

We got to the hospital around 11 PM. There was no one in the hospital birth center when we arrived, so they wheeled me to labor and delivery. (The contractions were too strong for me to walk at this point.) They had me laying on a stretcher in triage when I told the nurse, "I'm pretty sure this baby is coming now!" When I said that, she checked me, and said, "Oh yeah, that's the baby's head!" They then rushed me on the stretcher down to the birth center so that I could deliver the baby there. Once we got there, they had me move onto the bed. (I was laying on my side and had absolutely no desire or strength to move to a different position.) Once on the bed, I told the nurse that I needed to start pushing.

Ryan was there by my side the whole time, being amazing, trying to calm me down. I started a combination of breathing the baby out and pushing before the midwife and nurse arrived. They arrived fairly quickly after I started pushing. Everyone was awesome, reminding me to use my J breaths. I found that when they reminded me to groan (instead of screaming), everything went much smoother. They used a warm oil compress on my perineum, and with 4 or 5 contractions, I breathed/pushed the baby out (at 12:14 AM, just over 2 hours from the time my water broke). They immediately put him on my chest. Ryan was supposed to tell me the sex, but he was in such shock that there was a baby there, that I had to ask him what it was! He remarked, "it's a baby!" because he was so shocked by how quickly we went from watching a movie to becoming parents. Turned out it was Felix! They let him lay on my chest nursing for the next 2 or 3 hours before they weighed him (6 lbs 7 oz and 18 inches, although the doctor measured him at 19.5 inches a couple days later) and gave him the eye drops and Vitamin K injection. After the initial shock that we just had a baby wore off, we fell instantly in love with our little guy (and can't keep our eyes and hands off him now).

In summary, while I didn't have time to have the calm "Hypnobirthing" experience that I had planned and expected, I will definitely say that if I had not taken hypnobirthing, I don't think I would have been calm enough to make it through the labor like I did. The midwife and nurses said that I seemed so calm and asked if I had taken hypnobirthing, so maybe I was calmer than I felt. The whole experience was the craziest combination of being as physically in my body as possible while also being like an out of body experience. I definitely went inward. I had to ask Ryan after the birth how many people were in the room when I delivered Felix. I couldn't have told you if it was 2 or 50. I was that tuned into my own self. I loved my birth!!! Even though there were moments when I felt like I couldn't do it, there were also lots of moments where I felt like I could, and I did!

Oh, by the way, I didn't tear at all! That was the thing I was most scared of. I didn't have any pain meds before, during, or after the birth. The nurses and midwife seemed pretty impressed with how easily and quickly I recovered. I couldn't ask for a better birth experience! I already feel excited to be pregnant and go through all of this again! Little Felix is the most amazing thing I've ever seen. I can't believe how much I love him, and neither can Ryan. We are both stuck in a crazy tired state of euphoria.

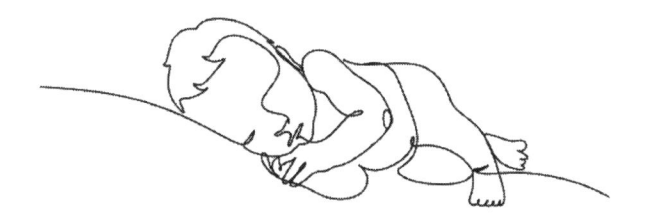

Eliza Lynn
Born November 13, 2013 at 6:57 PM
Birth story written December 3, 2013

It's been two weeks and six days since Eliza was born at home, in our bedroom, after the perfect birth experience. I'm still falling more and more in love with her every day, but I don't expect this to stop, ever. (I'm constantly amazed that I can love Felix more every day, and I know the same will happen with Eliza.) Before the time passes too much and I forget the details, here's her birth story.

I was 38 weeks pregnant, and I never thought I'd have made it that far. I had Felix at 36 weeks 3 days, and I had been having preterm labor symptoms this time around since about 30 weeks (almost constant Braxton Hicks, lost my mucus plug, etc.). So at 38 weeks, I was starting to feel like I was 42 weeks pregnant and I couldn't wait to meet this little one!

On Tuesday, November 12th, I left work feeling crampy. I picked up Felix from the babysitter's. He hadn't napped all day, so he fell asleep in the car. I carried him in and put him down on the couch, where he slept. I then called my sister and told her that I felt like I was going to have the baby. I was feeling very crampy still and having lots of Braxton Hicks contractions. She came over and we were both very excited about the possibility of me having the baby! I made dinner. We were eating when Felix woke up screaming and wouldn't stop. This stopped all crampy feelings I had and sent the baby shooting right back up into my uterus! That night, after we'd finally gotten Felix to sleep and then got in bed ourselves to watch an episode of *Parenthood*, I started timing the contractions I was having (still feeling like Braxton Hicks). They were coming seven minutes apart, which made me think that I'd be having the baby that night! I couldn't fall asleep for at least an hour because I was so excited. But eventually, I fell asleep.

    I woke up the next morning, November 13th, and got ready for work as usual. While I was making coffee and having breakfast, I kept having crampy-feeling contractions, and started to wonder if maybe I shouldn't go to work. But, the contractions were not in any way painful, so I went to work. While I was at work that day, I really felt like "today is the day!" I went out into the zoo (where I worked) but felt like I shouldn't walk all the way out there, so I asked my boss if I could take his golf cart, telling him that I thought I might have the baby today. He looked at me surprised, and asked if I was serious. I said I was serious, but that I needed to finish my work first! Haha!

Later that day, I sat through an all-employee meeting timing my contractions. My supervisor kept looking at me and saying, "Well???" while I was timing them. They weren't regular yet though, so I figured I still had time. After the meeting, I did a little more work, and then my colleagues and I went out to lunch. Even before we left, I felt like I was getting close to having a baby, but I needed to eat (it was already past 2 PM), so I decided to go to lunch anyway. While we were eating (falafel sandwich, carrot/beet juice, and lentil soup), my contractions started getting stronger and closer together. It was really a surreal experience, sitting there with colleagues while I was sure I was in labor and would have a baby any time! It was hard to talk or think of anything but the impending birth, but I tried! Towards the end of the meal, I started to really feel like I was in labor, so I ate hurriedly and then left to go have a baby!

I had been texting my midwife the night before and during the day giving her updates. So, on my way home, I called her and told her that I was pretty sure at this point that I was in labor. I told her I'd just had lunch with my boss and was on my way home. She asked how close my contractions were. When I told her that I hadn't been timing them, she asked me to time them for 15 minutes or so when I got home and then to call her back. I also called Ryan and told him to come home because I was having the baby!

When I got home (3:50 PM), I had to poop, and started timing my contractions while I was going to the bathroom. They were coming between three and four minutes apart, but still weren't in any way painful. I told my midwife that, and told her that I'd just had a bowel movement (sign of labor!), and she and her assistant got ready to come over. While I was waiting for them, my sister came over to help me get the house ready while we waited for Ryan and the midwives. There was definitely excitement in the air! I couldn't wait to meet this little one.

    I ran around for about 30 minutes making the bed and getting the herbal bath ready. The contractions kept coming, but they still weren't anything more than mildly uncomfortable. Ryan got home while we were getting things ready, and the midwife assistant arrived shortly after. I continued to stay busy getting things ready, and chatted with everyone as I did so. I was smiling and laughing, so she asked me if I was sure I was in labor. Ryan and I both assured her that this was how early labor was for me, and that things would pick up quickly. I am so incredibly lucky that my labors are so easy that the midwives don't even believe I'm in labor!

    Around 4:30, my midwife arrived. In the next 20 minutes or so, the contractions started to get more uncomfortable, causing me to have to stop and then to have to bend over and breathe deeply. But they were still very manageable. It was around that time that my midwife asked me if she could check my dilation, because she also wasn't really sure that I was very far along. I told her I'd rather she didn't check because I didn't want to be disappointed. So, she didn't check me.

    Around 5 PM, I started having more intense contractions that were progressively closer together (maybe

2 minutes apart) and required me to moan deeply. Luckily, the setting was perfect. We had all the candles lit in the bathroom and Indian classical music playing quietly. The lights were all dim. It was exactly how I imagined a home birth should be. Some time between 5 PM and 6 PM, I got in the bathtub and labored there (just Ryan and I) for about 45 minutes. Ryan was absolutely amazing the entire time. He used light touch massage on my back, put hot wash cloths on my lower back when needed, and just kept telling me how much he loved me and how amazing I was. It was perfect. He was my rock.

At one point, my midwife came into the bathroom and put gloves on. I think my moans were getting more intense, so she thought I was transitioning. But I was worried that she was just trying to trick me into thinking the baby was coming soon so that I wouldn't give up.

After laboring in the tub for a while, the contractions were becoming really intense and the water wasn't deep enough, so I got out and moved to the bedroom. The only way I felt comfortable was to be on my knees with my upper body laying on the bed. That's how I stayed until Eliza was born. Ryan says that I was in that position in the bedroom for about an hour. I feel like it was only 10 minutes, so who knows!

Either way, I stayed there, moaning like a cow, swearing only once, until it came time to push. All of this really felt like it took only a few minutes. Shortly before Eliza was born, my water finally broke! It shot out of me so hard I thought it was the baby! After that, I think I pushed two or three times, and Eliza was born at 6:57 PM! Ryan caught her, and then gave her to me, saying, "look at what it is!" I moved the umbilical cord out of the way and saw that it was a girl! And then I cried and cried...kneeling there on the floor in our own bedroom where this little girl was conceived, holding my precious little girl. I was so happy to meet her and so happy that labor was over! I looked down at her crying and told Ryan that this was Eliza! Within minutes, I was laying in bed nursing Eliza.

At around 9PM, my sister and brother-in-law brought Felix home to meet his new sister. He was instantly in love, calling her baby and kissing her. It was the sweetest moment of my life.

This labor was different from Felix's because I was so relaxed. After I got everything ready, I walked around feeling like I didn't know what to do! Several times while I was in the tub, I found myself clenching the tub with my fists, but then I told myself to just relax my entire body, and the contractions became so much more manageable! I never felt like I couldn't do it. Towards the end, I felt like I didn't WANT to do it anymore, but I knew that I could. Birth is so empowering, and home birth is even more so, because you are taking control of how your little one enters this world. I am so incredibly happy with both of my birth experiences. Having Felix in the birth center was perfect because he was my first. I would have panicked at the contractions if I had stayed home with him because I didn't know what to expect and I didn't know how long labor would last. But after the amazing experience of birthing Felix, I had the confidence necessary to have an amazing home birth with Eliza. And now I sit here wondering if I'll ever experience this again. Birth is such an amazing thing, and if it didn't mean lots of sleepless nights and if it was free to raise babies, we might end up with 20 of them because I love the process so much. But for now, I feel complete in our wonderful family of four. I couldn't be luckier.

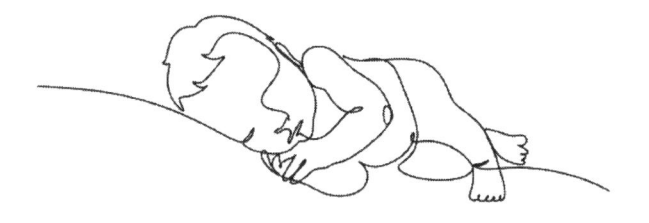

Fletcher Thomas
Born July 2, 2018 at 9:05 PM
Birth story written July 20, 2018

July 2 was a Monday, my first day home with the kids. The Friday before had been my last day at work. We had a great weekend. I needed to relax with the kids before this new soul could enter the world. On Sunday, we went to Belle Isle for a picnic and then to the splash pad on the riverfront. Then we made limeade at home. It was a wonderful day.

That Monday morning, Felix had a safety swimming class where Eliza and I were also allowed to participate and swim. My belly was huge in my bikini, but it felt great to be in the water, and to be spending time, just the three of us. After swimming, I noticed contractions with more pressure while we drove home. I didn't think much of them because I'd been having contractions since about 23 weeks. We came home and I made us quesadillas for lunch. While we ate, the contractions continued, but again, I didn't give them much weight. I had a case of the contraction who cried wolf. After lunch, I cleaned up and then we had quiet time.

During quiet time, I laid in my bed and timed my contractions. They were about six minutes apart and a minute long, but with more pressure. I started to think they were real so I sent my midwife a text at 3:30. Felix and Eliza had wanted to go to the library to get a book that was on hold (*Ook and Gluk*), so around 4 PM, we got ready and went to the library. Before we left, I called my sister and Ryan and told them they needed to come home. By that time, the contractions were between two and four minutes apart. They were getting more intense, but still very manageable.

Once we got to the library, I hurried the kids along while timing the contractions. It was quite the experience to know I was in labor while we were at the library. On the way home (4:18 PM), I called my midwife and told her that I thought she should come over. She jokingly told me that she felt like I was faking because I sounded normal. But, I knew that I was in labor. We talked and agreed that she would go to a prenatal in Sterling Heights and then head my way.

When we got home, I started to get everything ready. My sister showed up first, and started to take photos. The kids were very excited that the baby was on the way. Ryan got home soon after, and took a quick shower, before helping to fill up the birth pool. By 5:20, the contractions were two minutes apart and more intense. Around that time, I ate a bowl of cereal so that I wouldn't be too hungry. My midwives showed up soon after.

After they arrived, everything was already set up, so I vacuumed downstairs, taking breaks when a contraction came along. I was so sick of food sticking to my feet when I walked! They laughed. The atmosphere was quite joyful. I couldn't wait to meet this baby. The contractions continued to get more intense, but I could still just stop and breathe through them for a couple more hours. I got into the pool, but that was so relaxing that my contractions slowed, so I got out and walked up and down the stairs a few times to bring them closer together. Eventually, I got back into the pool.

Ryan and the kids were amazing at soothing me during contractions. We had to stop Felix from excitedly jumping around the birth pool. He couldn't wait. I got through a lot of the contractions by whispering to myself "this is temporary" over and over again. Ryan said he didn't know what I was saying and frantically tried to figure out what I was asking for every time I whispered! Telling myself that the pressure was temporary really helped me to get through those contractions.

My midwife told me that it was around 7:30 when I went into active labor. She said that's when I started vocalizing. I felt like I was so loud, groaning deeply, but she told me later that I was actually pretty quiet. I have no idea how close together those contractions were, or how long they lasted, but I remember feeling like they were coming one on top of the other, with little room to rest in between. I gripped onto the pool for a few, feeling out of control, but would then quickly release my grip and try to just be present in the moment, knowing that all of that incredible power in my uterus was bringing my baby closer to me. After about an hour and a half of those intense contractions, I started to feel like I couldn't do it anymore. I was transitioning.

At that time, my midwife encouraged me to feel for my baby. I can't remember if this was before or after I started pushing. I felt, and I could feel the head a few inches inside of my vagina. Once I felt that, I knew that the baby was almost here, and I used every ounce of strength to push that baby out of me. I think he went from a few inches inside of me to head out in one huge push! Then, on the next push, I pushed his body out and reached down into the water to grab him and pull him up. Oh, the relief at knowing that I was done, and that my baby was in my arms was incredible. I cried.

I don't know if I looked first, or if Ryan did, but somehow we then found out that it was a boy! I had given birth on my knees with my body draped over the edge of the pool. So I then sat back and brought my little guy to my chest. Ryan cried, and Felix and Eliza rushed over to meet their baby brother. My little guy, who didn't have a name yet, cried and cried. His lungs were so strong. Shortly after he was born, he bobbed his little head around, trying to find my breast. We talked then about his name. We had thought it would be Fletcher Thomas, but a few days before he was born I had a dream that I had a baby whose name was Gus. So I considered Gus. But Felix, Eliza, and Ryan were all set on Fletcher. I mulled it over for a few hours, and decided the next morning that this was indeed the Fletcher who had been out there, looking for us since Eliza was born. I feel so strongly connected to this little guy.

After a bit, I birthed the placenta. (Those contractions weren't fun because I just wanted to be done!)

Felix and Eliza looked at the placenta and remarked about how disgusting it was. But when I asked them about the birth, Felix said "I thought it was going to be scary, but it was just fun!" Eliza also really seemed to enjoy it. I then took an herbal bath and got in bed. After my midwives cleaned up and did the newborn exam, they left us around midnight and we all went to sleep.

The ultimate in power: surrendering when things don't go as planned

Are you wondering how you will feel if you prepare as I've suggested and birth doesn't go your way? You might be thinking that this sort of experience isn't possible for you. Maybe you are worried that allowing yourself to have such high expectations will leave you disappointed? There are women who do everything they can to prepare for an empowered, awakened birth, women who are ready to be transformed, but the stars don't align the way they had hoped, and maybe they end up with an emergency cesarean or a forceps delivery. Or maybe their baby needs extra care after they are born, and they aren't able to enjoy that golden hour of bonding. What I want you to know is that your preparation will not be for naught if you are one of the few who ends up needing the magic of Western medicine to help you and your baby. Instead, your preparation will allow you to surrender to the parts of birth that you didn't invite in, even if you don't fully want to, and trust in your provider that they truly have your best interest at heart.

While I look back on my birth experiences with so much gratitude, I myself experienced an unexpected turn very soon after Fletcher was born. What felt like a picture perfect birth experience was quickly overshadowed when we realized that he wasn't able to breathe well. Let me share the rest of his story with you now so that you can see that, even when things don't work out as planned, even when we have to surrender, there is still so much power in the love we have for our children. That power and that love bring us through birth and then bring us through even the toughest times so that we can transform and awaken into the very best versions of ourselves.

Fletcher's Birth: The Next Day (written when Fletcher was 18 days old)

The rest of this is hard for me to write. I'm not sure if I want to write it down or not. I'm still scared and heartbroken. But, here it goes. My hope is that this will be cathartic.

The next morning, Felix and Eliza woke at 6 AM, so excited to see their baby brother. Ryan made us cinnamon rolls and brought everything upstairs on trays. We were all exhausted but glowing in the love that this new baby boy brought to our family.

Around noon that day, we noticed that Fletcher's breathing was more labored than it should be. Ryan asked me if it was normal, and while at first I told him I thought it was, that he was just trying to get amniotic fluid out of his lungs, soon after I started to worry. I texted my midwife a video of him breathing, and she said it wasn't normal. She thought he might have transient tachypnea (a delay in the clearance of lung fluid that usually clears up on its own) and suggested a certain homeopathic remedy. My sister went and bought it for us and brought it over with some kombucha and chocolates. We gave it to him and thought we saw some improvement, but then we started to get worried again. My midwife said she would come over to do his 24-hour exam around 9 PM that night. When she did, she did a pulse ox test, and he failed. With that, and his labored breathing, she suggested that we take him into the hospital because the failed pulse ox test could be indicative of a heart abnormality. Tears started streaming down my face. I was heartbroken, and so terrified. We called my sister and asked her to come watch the kids so that we could take him to the hospital. She quickly came over; we gathered up some things in case we were admitted and left. Ryan asked me if he should speed. We were so worried.

When we arrived at the hospital, Ryan dropped me and Fletcher off at the doors and went and parked. I walked in with him, and they didn't make me go through the security. They knew something was wrong. Our midwife was waiting for me inside, and luckily, my oldest friend, who was a nurse at the hospital, was there too. She asked what was wrong and I cried that he wasn't breathing well. She took him from me and walked very quickly down the hall. My midwife and I followed. He looked over her shoulder at me. I felt helpless.

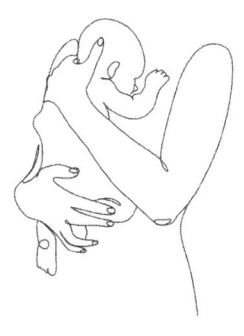

I find it incredibly ironic that I've just written a book about the power that you can find during birth, only to end my last birth story saying, "I felt helpless." Helplessness is clearly the opposite of power. And I did feel that. I went back and forth about whether I should include this part of my story, because it happened after the birth was over, and honestly, because the utter helplessness I felt when my baby was taken from my arms to the NICU doesn't fit with the feeling of empowerment. But when I thought more, and when I reflected on the weeks after that NICU stay and the power I found within me to care for a baby with special needs, night and day, I knew that I had unearthed the power necessary to be strong for Fletcher when I birthed him. And then I had used that power, the power of parenthood, to be fully present for what came next. I want you to know that power is not found only when things go your way. Instead, true power, the most earth-shaking power, can come when you prepare and then truly surrender and learn to trust. It was in those weeks that followed that my power transformed me.

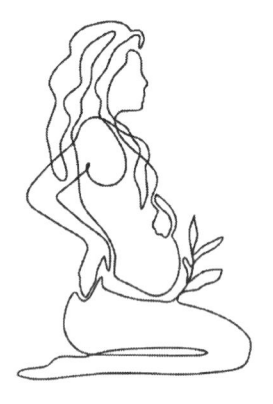

Conversation 10

The power of presence postpartum

I want to continue this story to show you how I found presence and transformation during those days after Fletcher's NICU stay. I'm writing the rest of his story now, because when I wrote his birth story, I didn't yet know how things would turn out. I didn't know if he'd need surgery or if he'd have trouble nursing or if he'd have breathing problems forever. I didn't know, but I pulled from that deep power inside of me, the power that brought me through three births, to be the very best mom I could be. Here's the rest of that story.

When my youngest was born, we spent the first day of his life listening to the squeakiness of his breathing, watching how each of his ribs became visible with each breath he took, and sending videos to our midwife, asking if this was normal. She came over that day and tested the amount of oxygen in his blood using a pulse oximeter. Our hearts sank when she told us he had failed this test, that his breathing was abnormal, and that we should take him to the emergency room immediately. I still remember how tiny he was in the car seat that evening, and how terrified I was on the drive there, worried that he might stop breathing at any moment. We rushed him into the ER, where my oldest friend (who is an ER nurse) waited, like my guardian angel. I still remember the look of anguish on her face as she saw my fear. She grabbed my baby from me, holding him upright, and ran him straight to the ER. I'm forever grateful that she was there with us at that moment.

I spent the next four days with my baby in the NICU, waiting for a diagnosis. I yearned to hold him for those first hours as he lay in an incubator hooked up to a breathing machine. And once I was permitted to hold him and nurse him, I didn't ever want to put him down again. After the longest four days of my life we found out that he had an airway disorder called laryngomalacia, and we were sent home with orders to return to the ear, nose, and throat specialist in a couple of weeks. They sent us home with a baby who struggled to breathe. He sounded like a dog's squeak toy, and the force it took him to take in air meant that his ribs stuck out with each breath.

For the next ten weeks, before he had surgery to correct his airway, my only job was to keep my baby alive. I was there to hold him in exactly the right position, the position that allowed him to breathe the quietest, while he slept. This, of course, meant that I barely slept. I was there to walk him around outside, as his terrified, wide open eyes looked up at me from the carrier I wore him in, as if he were asking me "Why, mama?!?!? Why can't I breathe?" But I stayed calm, and I walked him.

Finding Presence

During those ten weeks, I was exactly where I was meant to be in the world. The only place I was meant to be. Keeping my baby alive. Other than the times when I was on parental leave with my older two, this was the only time since becoming a parent when I found myself exactly where I wanted and needed to be. The rest of my parenting life has been spent working and feeling like I'm not with my kids enough or, ironically, home with my kids and feeling like I'm not working enough.

And in that space of presence, I began to experience the magic of the Universe. I think it is no accident that during a time when I was afraid for my son's life, I looked inward. I read Eckhart Tolle's *A New Earth* at this time, and it changed the way I live in the world. At a time when I had no choice but to be present in the moment, Eckhart was telling me that presence was the pathway to alleviating suffering. I sat with Fletcher sleeping on me while I read, purposely feeling the tingling of my hands and remarking on the beauty and absolute magic of the flowers and trees. (I hear you. I sound like I was doing some sort of psychedelic, but I wasn't. Read the book before you judge!) There was one moment (I'd call it an awakening if I didn't feel like that's somewhat self-aggrandizing), when I was on a walk across the street from my house with my older two kids, wearing the baby. It was a hot and humid summer day and we were standing under a tree with the most luscious green leaves. And quite suddenly, I felt myself having an intense sensory experience. It felt as if time slowed down as I remarked on the melodious laughter of my children and looked around at the jewel-tones of the trees and grass and flowers and sky. My skin marveled at the delicious heaviness of the hot, humid summer air. I felt like I was seeing the world *for the very first time*, as if through the eyes of a baby. I felt immense gratitude for everything that was happening in that moment. And having experienced that presence, my eyes were opened to the possibilities of life.

While it took me three tries with postpartum experiences and a baby who struggled to breathe to bring me to this moment of transformation, I feel that if I had known this was possible when I was younger, if I had known that I was exactly where I needed to be and had I marveled in the NOW, I would have been able to begin this journey of transformation even earlier. Of course, I may have scoffed at the idea as well. Maybe I wouldn't have been ready. And maybe you won't be ready either, but I want you to know that the presence you can achieve as the parent of a brand new baby is like no other time in your life. Use that time to transform your relationship with the present moment, to grow, and to more fully step into your power as a parent and a person.

I imagine you're wondering how. That's a really good question and I honestly don't have the exact recipe to begin the journey of inner awakening and empowerment. I can recommend tools like meditation, writing in a journal or morning pages (check out *The Artist's Way*), practicing gratitude, and seeking out the natural beauty in your world. Will these practices transform you? Maybe? Maybe not?

Regardless of whether you achieve some earth-shaking awakening, practices like these will surely ground you in the now and allow you to more easily and genuinely enjoy the most fleeting (but perhaps most amazing) time of life, when your child is a tiny baby. And that is the most important part of empowering yourself through birth and parenting: finding presence in the now. By doing that, you are disarming the power of the past and the future, stopping those times from impacting your now, and will be well on the way to living a fuller and more satisfying life.

Finding power in birth

For some of you, you might read this book and go through birth, only to find yourself wanting to send me a very angry letter telling me how painful your experience was and how I was wrong about birth. I want you to know now, before you go through birth, that every experience in life is unique to each person. And while I have research and my own lived experience to suggest that birth can be empowering, can help one to awaken, and that it does not have to be painful, I also know that it is hard work and that even with preparation, it may not go as planned. What I want for you if things don't go as planned is for you to go deep within yourself and find your power. I want you to know that even when birth is hard, (and even if you're cursing at me during a contraction that it is f#*%ing painful!), you are going through the most intense situation of your life so that you can bring a new human earthside. Even if you end up feeling like it's painful or using an epidural as a tool to make it through or having a cesarean, you are powerful because you are a portal for life.

I offer my stories not as the picture-perfect ideation of birth. Your birth story may look very different from my own. I offer my stories so that you can begin to see birth differently from the twisted tales the patriarchy has spun for us, convincing us all that birth is something our bodies are not capable of doing. We are animals. And just like our mammalian cousins, just like the squirrels in your yard, the deer in the forest, or the tigers in the jungles, our bodies were designed to bring new life into the world. And I cannot speak for the squirrels or the deer or the tigers regarding their states of consciousness surrounding birth, but I would not be surprised if their minds were also designed to be awakened, for consciousness to transform, as I believe ours do, when our hearts jump out of our bodies to become the hearts of our children, and we leap fearlessly into parenthood.

How do you want to use your power?

What will you do with the power that you unearth from deep in your uterus? As the last bit of preparation, before I leave you to meet your baby, I'd like you to journal on this. Talk it through. Imagine a new future for yourself where you are all the things you want to be. How would you live in the world? What kind of parent would you be? What kind of person would you be? Now is the time to envision a new future for you and your family, because if you can be the portal for new humans to enter the world, you can literally do anything you set your mind to. Go change the world and let me know how you are using your birth power.

www.awakenthrubirth.com
Instagram @awakenthrubirth

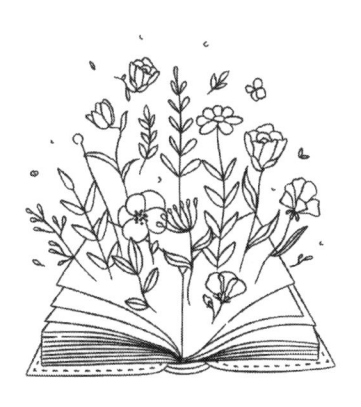

Recommended Resources to Learn More

Websites, Podcasts, and Apps

- Evidence-Based Birth—website and podcast–
  https://evidencebasedbirth.com
- The Birth Hour—podcast and their "Know Your Options" childbirth course–
  https://thebirthhour.com
- The Positive Birth Story Podcast–
  https://www.thepositivebirthstorypodcast.com/
- La Leche League–https://llli.org

Books

- Cameron, J. (2016). *The Artist's Way*. Penguin.
- Dispenza, J. (2013). *Breaking the habit of being yourself: How to lose your mind and create a new one*. Hay House, Inc.

- England, P., & Horowitz, R. (1998). *Birthing from within: An extra-ordinary guide to childbirth preparation* (No. Sirsi) i9780965987301). Albuquerque: Partera Press.
- Gaskin, I. M. (2010). *Spiritual Midwifery*. Book Publishing Company.
- Gaskin, I. M. (2011). *Birth Matters: A Midwife's Manifesta*. New York.
- Gaskin, I. M. (2003). *Ina May's Guide to Childbirth: Updated With New Material*. Bantam.
- Mongan, M. (2016). *HypnoBirthing: the Mongan Method*. Souvenir Press Limited.
- Tolle, E. (2006). *A New Earth: Awakening to your life's purpose*. Penguin Life.
- Tsabary, S. (2016). *The Awakened Family: A Revolution in Parenting*. Penguin.
- Wiessinger, Diane, Diana West, and Teresa Pitman. 2010. *The Womanly Art of Breastfeeding: Completely Revised and Updated 8th Edition*. Updated edition. Random House Publishing Group.

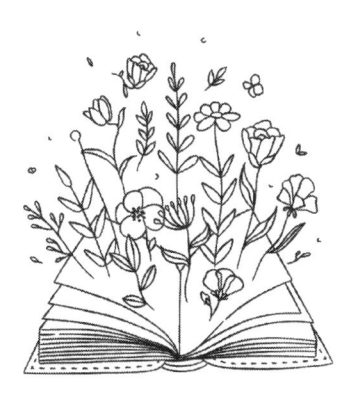

References

1. Gökçe İsbir, G., Yılmaz, M. & Thomson, G. Using an emotion-focused approach in preventing psychological birth trauma. *Perspect. Psychiatr. Care* **58**, 1170–1176 (2022).
2. Beck, C. T. & Watson, S. Impact of birth trauma on breastfeeding: a tale of two pathways. *Nurs. Res.* **57**, 228–236 (2008).
3. Uddin, N., Ayers, S., Khine, R. & Webb, R. The perceived impact of birth trauma witnessed by maternity health professionals: A systematic review. *Midwifery* **114**, 103460 (2022).
4. Kendall-Tackett, K. Birth Trauma: The Causes and Consequences of Childbirth-Related Trauma and PTSD. in *Women's Reproductive Mental Health Across the Lifespan* (ed. Barnes, D. L.) 177–191 (Springer International Publishing, 2014).
5. Shaban, Z. *et al.* Post-Traumatic Stress Disorder (PTSD) Following Childbirth: Prevalence and Contributing Factors. *Iran. Red Crescent Med. J.* **15**, 177–182 (2013).
6. Ayers, S., Wright, D. B. & Thornton, A. Development of a Measure of Postpartum PTSD: The City Birth Trauma Scale. *Front. Psychiatry* **9**, 409 (2018).
7. Kuch, K. & Cox, B. J. Symptoms of PTSD in 124 survivors of the

Holocaust. *Am. J. Psychiatry* **149**, 337–340 (1992).
8. Shelby, R. A., Golden-Kreutz, D. M. & Andersen, B. L. PTSD diagnoses, subsyndromal symptoms, and comorbidities contribute to impairments for breast cancer survivors. *J. Trauma. Stress* **21**, 165–172 (2008).
9. Bergman, H. E., Przeworski, A. & Feeny, N. C. Rates of Subthreshold PTSD Among U.S. Military Veterans and Service Members: A Literature Review. *Mil. Psychol.* **29**, 117–127 (2017).
10. Hall, R. T. *et al.* A breast-feeding assessment score to evaluate the risk for cessation of breast-feeding by 7 to 10 days of age. *J. Pediatr.* **141**, 659–664 (2002).
11. Nissen, E. *et al.* Different patterns of oxytocin, prolactin but not cortisol release during breastfeeding in women delivered by caesarean section or by the vaginal route. *Early Hum. Dev.* **45**, 103–118 (1996).
12. Dewey, K. G. Maternal and fetal stress are associated with impaired lactogenesis in humans. *J. Nutr.* **131**, 3012S–5S (2001).
13. Manhire, K. M., Hagan, A. E. & Floyd, S. A. A descriptive account of New Zealand mothers' responses to open-ended questions on their breast feeding experiences. *Midwifery* (2007).
14. Molloy, E., Biggerstaff, D. L. & Sidebotham, P. A phenomenological exploration of parenting after birth trauma: Mothers perceptions of the first year. *Women Birth* **34**, 278–287 (2021).
15. Suarez, G. L., Morales, S., Metcalf, K. & Pérez-Edgar, K. E. Perinatal complications are associated with social anxiety: Indirect effects through temperament. *Infant Child Dev.* **28**, (2019).
16. Hirshfeld-Becker, D. R. *et al.* Pregnancy complications associated with childhood anxiety disorders. *Depress. Anxiety* **19**, 152–162 (2004).
17. Valeri, B. O. *et al.* Neonatal Invasive Procedures Predict Pain Intensity at School Age in Children Born Very Preterm. *Clin. J. Pain* **32**, 1086–1093 (2016).
18. Chamberlain, D. *Babies Remember Birth: And Other Extraordinary Scientific Discoveries About the Mi.* (Ballantine Books, 1989).

19. Comeau, A. *et al.* Home birth integration into the health care systems of eleven international jurisdictions. *Birth* **45**, 311–321 (2018).
20. Maternal mortality ratio (modeled estimate, per 100,000 live births) - New Zealand. *World Bank Open Data* https://data.worldbank.org/indicator/SH.STA.MMRT?locations=NZ&most_recent_value_desc=false.
21. Births and Natality. https://www.cdc.gov/nchs/fastats/births.htm (2023).
22. Working Together to Reduce Black Maternal Mortality. https://www.cdc.gov/healthequity/features/maternal-mortality/index.html (2023).
23. Maternal mortality ratio. https://www.cia.gov/the-world-factbook/field/maternal-mortality-ratio/country-comparison.
24. Elaraby, S. *et al.* Behavioural factors associated with fear of litigation as a driver for the increased use of caesarean sections: a scoping review. *BMJ Open* **13**, e070454 (2023).
25. Rossignol, M., Chaillet, N., Boughrassa, F. & Moutquin, J.-M. Interrelations between four antepartum obstetric interventions and cesarean delivery in women at low risk: a systematic review and modeling of the cascade of interventions. *Birth* **41**, 70–78 (2014).
26. Lothian, J. A. Healthy Birth Practice #4: Avoid Interventions Unless They Are Medically Necessary. *J. Perinat. Educ.* **28**, 94–103 (2019).
27. Shurtz, I. Malpractice law, physicians' financial incentives, and medical treatment: How do they interact? *J. Law Econ.* **57**, 1–29 (2014).
28. Press Release: Top 82 U.S. Non Profit Hospitals. *Open The Books* https://www.openthebooks.com/press-release-top-82-us-non-profit-hospitals/.
29. Ofri, D. Why are Nonprofit Hospitals So Highly Profitable. *NY Times* (2020).
30. Health costs associated with pregnancy, childbirth, and postpartum care. *Peterson-KFF Health System Tracker*

https://www.healthsystemtracker.org/brief/health-costs-associated-with-pregnancy-childbirth-and-postpartum-care/ (2022).

31. Sakai-Bizmark, R. *et al.* Evaluation of Hospital Cesarean Delivery-Related Profits and Rates in the United States. *JAMA Netw Open* **4**, e212235 (2021).

32. Morris, T. C-Section Epidemic. *Contexts* **13**, 70–72 (2014).

33. WHO statement on caesarean section rates. https://www.who.int/publications/i/item/WHO-RHR-15.02 (2015).

34. Whitburn, L. Y., Jones, L. E., Davey, M.-A. & McDonald, S. The nature of labour pain: An updated review of the literature. *Women Birth* **32**, 28–38 (2019).

35. Whitburn, L. Y., Jones, L. E., Davey, M.-A. & Small, R. Women's experiences of labour pain and the role of the mind: an exploratory study. *Midwifery* **30**, 1029–1035 (2014).

36. Kinoshita, Y. *et al.* Healthy baby delivered vaginally from a brain-dead mother. *Acute Med Surg* **2**, 211–213 (2015).

37. Linton, S. J. & Shaw, W. S. Impact of Psychological Factors in the Experience of Pain. *Phys. Ther.* **91**, 700–711 (2011).

38. Wiech, K. Deconstructing the sensation of pain: The influence of cognitive processes on pain perception. *Science* **354**, 584–587 (2016).

39. Flink, I. K., Mroczek, M. Z., Sullivan, M. J. L. & Linton, S. J. Pain in childbirth and postpartum recovery: the role of catastrophizing. *Eur. J. Pain* **13**, 312–316 (2009).

40. Sim, X. L. J. *et al.* Association of pain catastrophizing and depressive states with multidimensional early labor pain assessment in nulliparous women having epidural analgesia - A secondary analysis. *J. Pain Res.* **14**, 3099–3107 (2021).

41. Soares, A. D. S. *et al.* Association of pain catastrophizing with the incidence and severity of acute and persistent perineal pain after natural childbirth: longitudinal cohort study. *Braz J Anesthesiol* **63**, 317–321 (2013).

42. Tan, H. S. *et al.* Perceived stress during labor and its association

with depressive symptomatology, anxiety, and pain catastrophizing. *Sci. Rep.* **11**, 17005 (2021).
43. Moskowitz, J. T. Good Feelings in the Midst of Chronic Pain. https://blogs.scientificamerican.com/observations/good-feelings-in-the-midst-of-chronic-pain/.
44. Deng, Y. *et al.* A comparison of maternal fear of childbirth, labor pain intensity and intrapartum analgesic consumption between primiparas and multiparas: A cross-sectional study. *International Journal of Nursing Sciences* **8**, 380–387 (2021).
45. Jameei-Moghaddam, M. The Relationship Between Women's Satisfaction with Personnel's Support During Labor, Fear of Childbirth, and Duration of Labor Stages. *Shiraz E-Medical* (2022).
46. Hanssen, M. M., Peters, M. L., Boselie, J. J. & Meulders, A. Can positive affect attenuate (persistent) pain? State of the art and clinical implications. *Curr. Rheumatol. Rep.* **19**, 80 (2017).
47. Fields, H. L. MIND on Pain: The Psychology of Pain. *Scientific American* doi:10.1038/scientificamericanmind0909-42.
48. Moseley, G. L. & Arntz, A. The context of a noxious stimulus affects the pain it evokes. *Pain* **133**, 64–71 (2007).
49. Gündüz, N., Üşen, A. & Aydin Atar, E. The Impact of Perceived Social Support on Anxiety, Depression and Severity of Pain and Burnout Among Turkish Females With Fibromyalgia. *Arch Rheumatol* **34**, 186–195 (2019).
50. Montoya, P., Larbig, W., Braun, C., Preissl, H. & Birbaumer, N. Influence of social support and emotional context on pain processing and magnetic brain responses in fibromyalgia. *Arthritis Rheum.* **50**, 4035–4044 (2004).
51. Flink, I. K., Mroczek, M. Z., Sullivan, M. J. & Linton, S. J. Pain in childbirth and postpartum recovery. *the role of catastrophizing.*
52. Alehagen, S., Wijma, B., Lundberg, U. & Wijma, K. Fear, pain and stress hormones during childbirth. *J. Psychosom. Obstet. Gynaecol.* **26**, 153–165 (2005).
53. Junge, C. *et al.* Labor pain in women with and without severe fear of childbirth: A population-based, longitudinal study. *Birth* **45**, 469–477 (2018).

54. Grünebaum, A., McCullough, L., Klein, R. & Chervenak, F. A. US midwife-attended hospital births are increasing while physician-attended hospital births are decreasing: 2003-2018. *Am. J. Obstet. Gynecol.* **223**, 460–461 (2020).

55. Barreto, T., Peterson, L. E., Petterson, S. & Bazemore, A. W. Family Physicians Practicing High-Volume Obstetric Care Have Recently Dropped by One-Half. *Am. Fam. Physician* **95**, 762 (2017).

56. Cullen, J. Family Physicians Ability to Perform Cesarean Sections Can Reduce Maternal and Infant Mortality. *Journal of the American Board of Family Medicine: JABFM* vol. 34 6–9 (2021).

57. *State Licensure of Certified Professional Midwives: Position Statement—April 2012*. http://narm.org/pdffiles/State-Licensure-of-CPMs2012.pdf (Revised October 2021).

58. Stjernholm, Y. V., Charvalho, P. da S., Bergdahl, O., Vladic, T. & Petersson, M. Continuous Support Promotes Obstetric Labor Progress and Vaginal Delivery in Primiparous Women - A Randomized Controlled Study. *Front. Psychol.* **12**, 582823 (2021).

59. Akbarzadeh, M., Masoudi, Z., Hadianfard, M. J., Kasraeian, M. & Zare, N. Comparison of the effects of maternal supportive care and acupressure (BL32 acupoint) on pregnant women's pain intensity and delivery outcome. *J. Pregnancy* **2014**, 129208 (2014).

60. Bohren, M. A., Hofmeyr, G. J., Sakala, C., Fukuzawa, R. K. & Cuthbert, A. Continuous support for women during childbirth. *Cochrane Database Syst. Rev.* **7**, CD003766 (2017).

61. Jukic, A. M., Baird, D. D., Weinberg, C. R., McConnaughey, D. R. & Wilcox, A. J. Length of human pregnancy and contributors to its natural variation. *Hum. Reprod.* **28**, 2848–2855 (2013).

62. Dekker, R. The Evidence on: Due Dates. https://evidencebasedbirth.com/evidence-on-due-dates/ (2019)

63. Declercq, E. R., Sakala, C., Corry, M. P., Applebaum, S. & Herrlich, A. Major Survey Findings of Listening to Mothers(SM) III: Pregnancy and Birth: Report of the Third National U.S. Survey of Women's Childbearing Experiences. *J. Perinat. Educ.* **23**, 9–16 (2014).

64. Labor Induction. https://www.acog.org/womens-health/faqs/labor-induction.
65. Grobman, W. LB01: A randomized trial of elective induction of labor at 39 weeks compared with expectant management of low-risk nulliparous women. *Am. J. Obstet. Gynecol.* **218**, S601 (2018).
66. Hamm, R. F., Srinivas, S. K. & Levine, L. D. Risk factors and racial disparities related to low maternal birth satisfaction with labor induction: a prospective, cohort study. *BMC Pregnancy Childbirth* **19**, 530 (2019).
67. Shetty, A., Burt, R., Rice, P. & Templeton, A. Women's perceptions, expectations and satisfaction with induced labour—A questionnaire-based study. *Eur. J. Obstet. Gynecol. Reprod. Biol.* **123**, 56–61 (2005).
68. Coates, R., Cupples, G., Scamell, A. & McCourt, C. Women's experiences of induction of labour: Qualitative systematic review and thematic synthesis. *Midwifery* **69**, 17–28 (2019).
69. Johnson, K. C. & Daviss, B.-A. Outcomes of planned home births with certified professional midwives: large prospective study in North America. *BMJ* **330**, 1416 (2005).
70. Hutton, E. K., Reitsma, A. H. & Kaufman, K. Outcomes associated with planned home and planned hospital births in low-risk women attended by midwives in Ontario, Canada, 2003--2006: A retrospective cohort study. *Birth* **36**, 180–189 (2009).
71. Dekker, R. & Bertone, A. How often are providers inducing for due dates? https://evidencebasedbirth.com/evidence-on-inducing-labor-for-going-past-your-due-date/ (2020)
72. Friedman, E. A. Primigravid labor; a graphicostatistical analysis. *Obstet. Gynecol.* **6**, 567–589 (1955).
73. Safe Prevention of the Primary Cesarean Delivery. https://www.acog.org/clinical/clinical-guidance/obstetric-care-consensus/articles/2014/03/safe-prevention-of-the-primary-cesarean-delivery.
74. Wilson, R. D. I. A. The Evidence on: Friedman's Curve and Failure to Progress: A Leading Cause of Unplanned Cesareans. https://evidencebasedbirth.com/friedmans-curve-and-failure-to-

progress-a-leading-cause-of-unplanned-c-sections/ (2022).
75. Alrais, M. A. *et al.* Adherence to Consensus Guidelines for the Management of Labor Arrest Disorders in a Single Academic Tertiary Care Medical Center. *Am. J. Perinatol.* **36**, 911–917 (2019).
76. Lothian, J. A., Amis, D. & Crenshaw, J. Care practice #4: no routine interventions. *J. Perinat. Educ.* **16**, 29–34 (2007).
77. Decker, R. & Bertone, A. The Evidence on: Fetal Monitoring. *Evidence-Based Birth* https://evidencebasedbirth.com/fetal-monitoring/ (2018).
78. Heelan-Fancher, L. *et al.* Impact of continuous electronic fetal monitoring on birth outcomes in low-risk pregnancies. *Birth* **46**, 311–317 (2019).
79. Paterno, M. T., McElroy, K. & Regan, M. Electronic Fetal Monitoring and Cesarean Birth: A Scoping Review. *Birth* **43**, 277–284 (2016).
80. Alfirevic, Z., Devane, D., Gyte, G. M. & Cuthbert, A. Continuous cardiotocography (CTG) as a form of electronic fetal monitoring (EFM) for fetal assessment during labour. *Cochrane Database Syst. Rev.* **2**, CD006066 (2017).
81. Approaches to Limit Intervention During Labor and Birth. https://www.acog.org/clinical/clinical-guidance/committee-opinion/articles/2019/02/approaches-to-limit-intervention-during-labor-and-birth.
82. Zang, Y. *et al.* Effects of flexible sacrum positions during the second stage of labour on maternal and neonatal outcomes: A systematic review and meta-analysis. *J. Clin. Nurs.* **29**, 3154–3169 (2020).
83. Berta, M., Lindgren, H., Christensson, K., Mekonnen, S. & Adefris, M. Effect of maternal birth positions on duration of second stage of labor: systematic review and meta-analysis. *BMC Pregnancy Childbirth* **19**, 1–8 (2019).
84. Dekker, R. The Evidence on: Birthing Positions. https://evidencebasedbirth.com/evidence-birthing-positions/ (2022).

85. Dundes, L. The evolution of maternal birthing position. *Am. J. Public Health* **77**, 636–641 (1987).
86. Adams, S. S., Eberhard-Gran, M. & Eskild, A. Fear of childbirth and duration of labour: a study of 2206 women with intended vaginal delivery. *BJOG* **119**, 1238–1246 (2012).
87. Bowman, L. Cervical reversal/regression. *Midwifery Matters* **108**, 14 (2006).
88. Daviss, B.-A. & Johnson, K. Departing from straightline obstetrics and timelines. https://understandingbirthbetter.com/UsingPlateausforUnderstandingbirthbetter_5.pdf.
89. Hodnett, E. D., Gates, S., Hofmeyr, G. J. & Sakala, C. Continuous support for women during childbirth. *Cochrane Database Syst. Rev.* **10**, CD003766 (2012).
90. Caughey, A. B., Cahill, A. G., Guise, J.-M. & Rouse, D. J. Safe prevention of the primary cesarean delivery. *Am. J. Obstet. Gynecol.* **210**, 179–193 (2014).
91. Fortier, J. H. & Godwin, M. Doula support compared with standard care: Meta-analysis of the effects on the rate of medical interventions during labour for low-risk women delivering at term. *Can. Fam. Physician* **61**, e284–e292 (2015).
92. Yang, J. & Bai, H. Knowledge, attitude and experience of episiotomy practice among obstetricians and midwives: a cross-sectional study from China. *BMJ Open* **11**, e043596 (2021).
93. What is an episiotomy? https://www.acog.org/womens-health/experts-and-stories/ask-acog/what-is-an-episiotomy.
94. Castlight Health, The Leapfrog Group. *Maternity Care: Data by hospital on nationally reported metrics.* https://www.leapfroggroup.org/sites/default/files/Files/leapfrog_castlight_maternity_care_2018%20report.pdf (2018).
95. Search Leapfrog's Hospital and Surgery Center Ratings. *Hospital and Surgery Center Ratings | Leapfrog Group* https://ratings.leapfroggroup.org/.
96. GHO | By category | Births by caesarean section - Data by country.

97. Cheyney, M. *et al.* Outcomes of care for 16,924 planned home births in the United States: the Midwives Alliance of North America Statistics Project, 2004 to 2009. *J. Midwifery Womens. Health* **59**, 17–27 (2014).
98. Cesarean Birth. https://www.acog.org/womens-health/faqs/cesarean-birth.
99. Costa-Ramón, A., Kortelainen, M., Rodríguez-González, A. & Sääksvuori, L. The Long-Run Effects of Cesarean Sections. *J. Hum. Resour.* **57**, 2048–2085 (2022).
100. Cheng, Y. W. *et al.* Litigation in obstetrics: does defensive medicine contribute to increases in cesarean delivery? *J. Matern. Fetal. Neonatal Med.* **27**, 1668–1675 (2014).
101. Montoya-Williams, D. *et al.* What Are Optimal Cesarean Section Rates in the U.S. and How Do We Get There? A Review of Evidence-Based Recommendations and Interventions. *J. Womens. Health* **26**, 1285–1291 (2017).
102. Delayed Umbilical Cord Clamping After Birth. https://www.acog.org/clinical/clinical-guidance/committee-opinion/articles/2020/12/delayed-umbilical-cord-clamping-after-birth.
103. *Position Statement: Optimal Management of the Umbilical Cord at the Time of Birth*. https://www.midwife.org/acnm/files/acnmlibrarydata/uploadfilename/000000000290/Optimal%20Management%202021_Final.pdf (2021).
104. Blix, E., Kumle, M., Kjærgaard, H., Øian, P. & Lindgren, H. E. Transfer to hospital in planned home births: a systematic review. *BMC Pregnancy Childbirth* **14**, 179 (2014).
105. Luce, A. *et al.* 'Is it realistic?' the portrayal of pregnancy and childbirth in the media. *BMC Pregnancy Childbirth* **16**, 40 (2016).
106. Shaw, D. *et al.* Drivers of maternity care in high-income countries: can health systems support woman-centred care? *Lancet* **388**, 2282–2295 (2016).
107. Lenhard, M. S. *et al.* Pelvimetry revisited: analyzing cephalopelvic disproportion. *Eur. J. Radiol.* **74**, e107–11 (2010).

108. Cephalopelvic Disproportion. *Cleveland Clinic* https://my.clevelandclinic.org/health/diseases/24466-cephalopelvic-disproportion.
109. Lederman, R. P., Lederman, E., Work, B. A. & McCann, D. S. The relationship of maternal anxiety, plasma catecholamines, and plasma cortisol to progress in labor. *Am. J. Obstet. Gynecol.* **132**, 495–500 (1978).
110. Jiang, H., Qian, X., Carroli, G. & Garner, P. Selective versus routine use of episiotomy for vaginal birth. *Cochrane Database Syst. Rev.* **2**, CD000081 (2017).
111. Smith, L. A., Price, N., Simonite, V. & Burns, E. E. Incidence of and risk factors for perineal trauma: a prospective observational study. *BMC Pregnancy Childbirth* **13**, 59 (2013).
112. Mongan, M. *HypnoBirthing, Fourth Edition: The breakthrough natural approach to safer, easier, more comfortable birthing - The Mongan Method, 4th Edition.* (Simon and Schuster, 2015).
113. Suzuki, S. Clinical significance of precipitous labor. *J. Clin. Med. Res.* **7**, 150–153 (2015).
114. Zhang, J. *et al.* Contemporary patterns of spontaneous labor with normal neonatal outcomes. *Obstet. Gynecol.* **116**, 1281–1287 (2010).
115. Dwiarini, M., Chou, H. F., Gau, M. L. & Liu, C. Y. Relationship between fear of childbirth, self-efficacy, and length of labor among nulliparous women in Indonesia. *Midwifery* (2022).
116. Koss, J., Bidzan, M., Smutek, J. & Bidzan, L. Influence of Perinatal Depression on Labor-Associated Fear and Emotional Attachment to the Child in High-Risk Pregnancies and the First Days After Delivery. *Med. Sci. Monit.* **22**, 1028–1037 (2016).
117. Cahill, H. A. Male appropriation and medicalization of childbirth: an historical analysis. *J. Adv. Nurs.* **33**, 334–342 (2001).
118. Nove, A., Berrington, A. & Matthews, Z. Comparing the odds of postpartum haemorrhage in planned home birth against planned hospital birth: results of an observational study of over 500,000 maternities in the UK. *BMC Pregnancy Childbirth* **12**, 130 (2012).
119. Bienstock, J. L., Eke, A. C. & Hueppchen, N. A. Postpartum Hemorrhage. *N. Engl. J. Med.* **384**, 1635–1645 (2021).

120. Corbetta-Rastelli, C. M. *et al.* Postpartum Hemorrhage Trends and Outcomes in the United States, 2000-2019. *Obstet. Gynecol.* **141**, 152–161 (2023).
121. Branjerdporn, G., Meredith, P., Wilson, T. & Strong, J. Prenatal Predictors of Maternal-infant Attachment. *Can. J. Occup. Ther.* **87**, 265–277 (2020).
122. Yazici, E., Kirkan, T. S., Aslan, P. A., Aydin, N. & Yazici, A. B. Untreated depression in the first trimester of pregnancy leads to postpartum depression: high rates from a natural follow-up study. *Neuropsychiatr. Dis. Treat.* **11**, 405–411 (2015).
123. Bauman, B. L. *et al.* Vital Signs: Postpartum Depressive Symptoms and Provider Discussions About Perinatal Depression - United States, 2018. *MMWR Morb. Mortal. Wkly. Rep.* **69**, 575–581 (2020).
124. Nillni, Y. I., Mehralizade, A., Mayer, L. & Milanovic, S. Treatment of depression, anxiety, and trauma-related disorders during the perinatal period: A systematic review. *Clin. Psychol. Rev.* **66**, 136–148 (2018).
125. Zappas, M. P., Becker, K. & Walton-Moss, B. Postpartum Anxiety. *J. Nurse Pract.* **17**, 60–64 (2021).
126. Tolle, E. *A New Earth: Awakening to Your Life's Purpose*. (Penguin Publishing Group, 2006).
127. Tsabary, S. *The Awakened Family: A Revolution in Parenting*. (Penguin, 2016).
128. Critcher, C. R. & Dunning, D. Self-affirmations provide a broader perspective on self-threat. *Pers. Soc. Psychol. Bull.* **41**, 3–18 (2015).
129. Cooke, R., Trebaczyk, H., Harris, P. & Wright, A. J. Self-affirmation promotes physical activity. *J. Sport Exerc. Psychol.* **36**, 217–223 (2014).
130. Epton, T. & Harris, P. R. Self-affirmation promotes health behavior change. *Health Psychol.* **27**, 746–752 (2008).
131. Layous, K. *et al.* Feeling left out, but affirmed: Protecting against the negative effects of low belonging in college. *J. Exp. Soc. Psychol.* **69**, 227–231 (2017).

132. Koole, S. L., Smeets, K., van Knippenberg, A. & Dijksterhuis, A. The cessation of rumination through self-affirmation. *J. Pers. Soc. Psychol.* **77**, 111–125 (1999).
133. Cascio, C. N. *et al.* Self-affirmation activates brain systems associated with self-related processing and reward and is reinforced by future orientation. *Soc. Cogn. Affect. Neurosci.* **11**, 621–629 (2016).
134. Rahayu, E. P. & Rizki, L. K. The Effect of Positive Affirmations to Anxiety level and 2nd stage of labor length. *sjik* **9**, 900–905 (2020).
135. Kasawara, K. T., do Nascimento, S. L., Costa, M. L., Surita, F. G. & e Silva, J. L. P. Exercise and physical activity in the prevention of pre-eclampsia: systematic review. *Acta Obstet. Gynecol. Scand.* **91**, 1147–1157 (2012).
136. Davenport, M. H. *et al.* Prenatal exercise for the prevention of gestational diabetes mellitus and hypertensive disorders of pregnancy: a systematic review and meta-analysis. *Br. J. Sports Med.* **52**, 1367–1375 (2018).
137. Hegaard, H. K., Pedersen, B. K., Nielsen, B. B. & Damm, P. Leisure time physical activity during pregnancy and impact on gestational diabetes mellitus, pre-eclampsia, preterm delivery and birth weight: a review. *Acta Obstet. Gynecol. Scand.* **86**, 1290–1296 (2007).
138. Ghandali, N. Y., Iravani, M., Habibi, A. & Cheraghian, B. The effectiveness of a Pilates exercise program during pregnancy on childbirth outcomes: a randomised controlled clinical trial. *BMC Pregnancy Childbirth* **21**, 480 (2021).
139. Bolanthakodi, C., Raghunandan, C., Saili, A., Mondal, S. & Saxena, P. Prenatal Yoga: Effects on Alleviation of Labor Pain and Birth Outcomes. *J. Altern. Complement. Med.* **24**, 1181–1188 (2018).
140. Barakat, R., Franco, E., Perales, M., López, C. & Mottola, M. F. Exercise during pregnancy is associated with a shorter duration of labor. A randomized clinical trial. *Eur. J. Obstet. Gynecol. Reprod. Biol.* **224**, 33–40 (2018).

141. Ulfsdottir, H., Saltvedt, S. & Georgsson, S. Women's experiences of waterbirth compared with conventional uncomplicated births. *Midwifery* **79**, 102547 (2019).
142. Lathrop, A., Bonsack, C. F. & Haas, D. M. Women's experiences with water birth: A matched groups prospective study. *Birth* **45**, 416–423 (2018).
143. Vanderlaan, J., Hall, P. J. & Lewitt, M. Neonatal outcomes with water birth: A systematic review and meta-analysis. *Midwifery* **59**, 27–38 (2018).
144. Cluett, E. R., Burns, E. & Cuthbert, A. Immersion in water during labour and birth. *Cochrane Database Syst. Rev.* **5**, CD000111 (2018).
145. Shaw-Battista, J. Systematic Review of Hydrotherapy Research. *J. Perinat. Neonatal Nurs.* **31**, 303–316 (2017).
146. Field, T., Hemandez-Reif, M., Taylor, S., Quintino, O. & Burman, I. Labor pain is reduced by massage therapy. *Journal of Psychosomatic Obstetrics & Gynecology* **18**, 286–291 (1997).
147. Taghinejad, H., Delpisheh, A. & Suhrabi, Z. Comparison between massage and music therapies to relieve the severity of labor pain. *Womens. Health* **6**, 377–381 (2010).
148. Field, T. Pregnancy and labor massage. *Expert Rev. Obstet. Gynecol.* **5**, 177–181 (2010).
149. Hosseini, S. E., Bagheri, M. & Honarparvaran, N. Investigating the effect of music on labor pain and progress in the active stage of first labor. *Eur. Rev. Med. Pharmacol. Sci.* **17**, 1479–1487 (2013).
150. Phumdoung, S. & Good, M. Music reduces sensation and distress of labor pain. *Pain Manag. Nurs.* **4**, 54–61 (2003).
151. Santiváñez-Acosta, R., Tapia-López, E. de L. N. & Santero, M. Music Therapy in Pain and Anxiety Management during Labor: A Systematic Review and Meta-Analysis. *Medicina* **56**, (2020).
152. Pérez-Aranda, A. *et al.* Laughing away the pain: A narrative review of humour, sense of humour and pain. *Eur. J. Pain* **23**, 220–233 (2019).
153. Stuber, M. *et al.* Laughter, humor and pain perception in children: a pilot study. *Evid. Based. Complement. Alternat. Med.* **6**,

271–276 (2009).
154. Chooi, C. S. L., Nerlekar, R., Raju, A. & Cyna, A. M. The effects of positive or negative words when assessing postoperative pain. *Anaesth. Intensive Care* **39**, 101–106 (2011).
155. Phillips, R. The Sacred Hour: Uninterrupted Skin-to-Skin Contact Immediately After Birth. *Newborn Infant Nurs. Rev.* **13**, 67–72 (2013).
156. Widström, A.-M., Brimdyr, K., Svensson, K., Cadwell, K. & Nissen, E. Skin-to-skin contact the first hour after birth, underlying implications and clinical practice. *Acta Paediatr.* **108**, 1192–1204 (2019).
157. Moore, E. R., Bergman, N. & Anderson, G. C. Early skin-to-skin contact for mothers and their healthy newborn infants. *of systematic Reviews* (2016).
158. Dekker, R. & Bertone, A. Evidence on: Pitocin® During the Third Stage of Labor. *Evidence-Based Birth* https://evidencebasedbirth.com/evidence-on-pitocin-during-the-third-stage-of-labor/ (2020).

@AWAKENTHRUBIRTH

Made in the USA
Columbia, SC
18 August 2023